T0228989

Early Diagnosis and Intervention in Predementia Alzheimer's Disease

Editors

JOSÉ L. MOLINUEVO
JEFFREY L. CUMMINGS
BRUNO DUBOIS
PHILIP SCHELTENS

MEDICAL CLINICS OF NORTH AMERICA

www.medical.theclinics.com

May 2013 • Volume 97 • Number 3

ELSEVIER

1600 John F. Kennedy Boulevard • Suite 1800 • Philadelphia, Pennsylvania, 19103-2899

http://www.theclinics.com

MEDICAL CLINICS OF NORTH AMERICA Volume 97, Number 3
May 2013 ISSN 0025-7125, ISBN-13: 978-1-4557-7117-2

Editor: Pamela Hetherington

Medical Clinics of North America (ISSN 0025-7125) is published bimonthly by Elsevier Inc., 360 Park Avenue South, New York, NY 10010-1710. Months of issue are January, March, May, July, September, and November. Periodicals postage paid at New York, NY, and additional mailing offices. Subscription prices are USD 241 per year for US individuals, USD 441 per year for US institutions, USD 121 per year for US students, USD 307 per year for Canadian individuals, USD 572 per year for Canadian institutions, USD 190 per year for Canadian students, USD 372 per year for international individuals, USD 572 per year for international institutions and USD 190 per year for international students. To receive student/resident rate, orders must be accompanied by name of affiliated institution, date of term, and the *signature* of program/residency coordinator on institution letterhead. Orders will be billed at individual rate until proof of status is received. Foreign air speed delivery is included in all *Clinics* subscription prices. All prices are subject to change without notice. **POSTMASTER:** Send address changes to *Medical Clinics of North America*, Elsevier Health Sciences Division, Subscription Customer Service, 3251 Riverport Lane, Maryland Heights, MO 63043. **Customer Service: Telephone: 1-800-654-2452** (U.S. and Canada); **1-314-447-8871** (outside U.S. and Canada). **Fax: 1-314-447-8029. E-mail: journalscustomerservice-usa@elsevier.com** (for print support); **journalsonlinesupport-usa@elsevier.com** (for online support).

Reprints. For copies of 100 or more of articles in this publication, please contact the Commercial Reprints Department, Elsevier Inc., 360 Park Avenue South, New York, NY 10010-1710. Tel.: 212-633-3812; Fax: 212-462-1935; E-mail: reprints@elsevier.com.

Medical Clinics of North America is also published in Spanish by McGraw-Hill Interamericana Editores S. A., P.O. Box 5-237, 06500 Mexico, D.F., Mexico.

Medical Clinics of North America is covered in *MEDLINE/PubMed (Index Medicus), Current Contents, ASCA, Excerpta Medica, Science Citation Index,* and *ISI/BIOMED.*

Printed and bound by CPI Group (UK) Ltd, Croydon, CR0 4YY

Transferred to digital print 2013

PROGRAM OBJECTIVE
The goal of the *Medical Clinics of North America* is to keep practicing physicians up to date with current clinical practice by providing timely articles reviewing the state of the art in patient care.

TARGET AUDIENCE
All practicing physicians and other healthcare professionals.

LEARNING OBJECTIVES
Upon completion of this activity, participants will be able to:
1. Review the emotional and psychological implications of early Alzheimer's Disease (AD) diagnosis.
2. Discuss the application of CSF Biomarkers and cognitive approaches to early AD diagnosis.
3. Describe clinical trials in predementia stages of AD.

ACCREDITATION
The Elsevier Office of Continuing Medical Education (EOCME) is accredited by the Accreditation Council for Continuing Medical Education (ACCME) to provide continuing medical education for physicians.

The EOCME designates this journal-based CME activity for a maximum of 9 *AMA PRA Category 1 Credit(s)*™. Physicians should claim only the credit commensurate with the extent of their participation in the activity.

All other health care professionals completing continuing education credit for this activity will be issued a certificate of participation.

DISCLOSURE OF CONFLICTS OF INTEREST
The EOCME assesses conflict of interest with its instructors, faculty, planners, and other individuals who are in a position to control the content of CME activities. All relevant conflicts of interest that are identified are thoroughly vetted by EOCME for fair balance, scientific objectivity, and patient care recommendations. EOCME is committed to providing its learners with CME activities that promote improvements or quality in healthcare and not a specific proprietary business or a commercial interest.

The planning committee, staff, authors and editors listed below have identified no financial relationships or relationships to products or devices they or their spouse/life partner have with commercial interest related to the content of this CME activity:
Pascal Antoine, PhD; Jessica Chew, BS; Francesco G. Garaci, PhD; Michel Grothe, PhD; Simone Lista, PhD; Jagan A. Pillai, MBBS, PhD; Lorena Rami, PhD; Philip Scheltens, MD, PhD; Stefan J. Teipel, Prof, Dr.; Nicola Toschi, PhD; Victor L. Villemange, MD; and Henrik Zetterberg, MD, PhD.

The planning committee, staff, authors and editors listed below have identified financial relationships or relationships to products or devices they or their spouse/life partner have with commercial interest related to the content of this CME activity:
Kaj Blennow, MD, PhD is a consultant/advisor for Innogenetics, Roche, Lilly and Pfizer.
Jeffrey L. Cummings, MD is a consultant for General Electric and Lilly; has a research grant from Avid.
Bruno Dubois, MD has a research grant from Pfizer.
Harald Hampel, MD is a consultant/advisor for Jung-Diagnostics, GE Healthcare and Avid.
John Harrison, C.Sci, C.Psychol is a consultant/advisor for Astra-Zeneca, Boehringer Ingleheim, Bracket (Clinical), CRF Health, EnVivo Pharma, EPharmaSolutions, Eisai, Eli Lilly, Janssen AI, Lundbeck, Med-Avante, Merck, MyCog, Novartis, Nutricia, Orion Pharma, Pharmanet/i3, Pfizer, Prana Biotech, Reviva, Servier, Shire, TCG, TransTech Pharma and Velacor.
José L. Molinuevo, MD, PhD is a consultant/advisor for Pfizer, MSD, Merz, Novartis, Lundbeck, Roche, Bayer, Bristol-Myers Squibb, GE Health Care, Lilly and Innogenetics.
Florence Pasquier, MD, PhD is a consultant/advisor for Lilly-Avid, Novartis and Nutricia.
Christopher C. Rowe, MD is on Speakers Bureau, is a consultant/advisor, and has a research grant for GE Healthcare, has a research grant from Avid/Lily Pharmaceuticals, Astra Zeneca and Bayer.
Daniel Silverman, MD, PhD is co-inventor of NeuroQ, licensed by Univ. of CA to SynterMed.

UNAPPROVED/OFF-LABEL USE DISCLOSURE
The EOCME requires CME faculty to disclose to the participants:
1. When products or procedures being discussed are off-label, unlabelled, experimental, and/or investigational (not US Food and Drug Administration (FDA) approved); and
2. Any limitations on the information presented, such as data that are preliminary or that represent ongoing research, interim analyses, and/or unsupported opinions. Faculty may discuss information about

pharmaceutical agents that is outside of FDA-approved labelling. This information is intended solely for CME and is not intended to promote off-label use of these medications. If you have any questions, contact the medical affairs department of the manufacturer for the most recent prescribing information.

TO ENROLL

To enroll in the *Medical Clinics of North America* Continuing Medical Education program, call customer service at 1-800-654-2452 or sign up online at http://www.theclinics.com/home/cme. The CME program is available to subscribers for an additional annual fee of USD $267.

METHOD OF PARTICIPATION

In order to claim credit, participants must complete the following:

1. Complete enrolment as indicated above.
2. Read the activity.
3. Complete the CME Test and Evaluation. Participants must achieve a score of 70% on the test. All CME Tests and Evaluations must be completed online.

CME INQUIRIES/SPECIAL NEEDS

For all CME inquiries or special needs, please contact elsevierCME@elsevier.com.

MEDICAL CLINICS OF NORTH AMERICA

FORTHCOMING ISSUES

July 2013
The Diabetic Foot
Andrew Boulton, *Editor*

September 2013
Infectious Disease Threats
Douglas Paauw, *Editor*

November 2013
Pre-Operative Management of the Patient with Chronic Disease
Jeffrey Kirsch, and Ansgar Brambrink, *Editors*

RECENT ISSUES

March 2013
Management of Acute and Chronic Headache Pain
Steven D. Waldman, MD, JD, *Editor*

January 2013
Diabetic Chronic Kidney Disease
Mark E. Williams, MD, FACP, FASN, *Editor*

November 2012
Interventions in Infectious Disease Emergencies
Nancy Misri Khardori, MD, PhD, FACP, FIDSA, *Editor*

RELATED INTEREST

Neuroimaging Clinics of North America Volume 22, Issue 4 (February 2012)
Imaging in Alzheimer's Disease and Other Dementias
Alison D. Murray, *Editor*

Contributors

EDITORS

JOSÉ L. MOLINUEVO, MD, PhD
Neurology Service, Alzheimer's Disease and Other Cognitive Disorders Unit, Hospital Clínic; Institut d'Investigació Biomédica August Pi I Sunyer (Neurodegenerative Diseases Group); ICN Hospital Clinic i Universitari and Pasqual Maragall Foundation, Barcelona, Spain

JEFFREY L. CUMMINGS, MD, ScD
Director, Lou Ruvo Center for Brain Health in Las Vegas, Andrea and Joseph Hahn Chair of Neurological Institute, Cleveland Clinic, Las Vegas, Nevada

BRUNO DUBOIS, MD
Fédération de Neurologie, Hôpital de la Salpêtrière, Paris, France

PHILIP SCHELTENS, MD
Professor of Cognitive Neurology, Director of the Alzheimer Center, VU University Medical Center, Amsterdam, Netherlands

AUTHORS

PASCAL ANTOINE, PhD
Professor, University Lille Nord de France, Lille; UDL3, URECA, Villeneuve d'Ascq, France

KAJ BLENNOW, MD, PhD
Clinical Neurochemistry Laboratory, Institute of Neuroscience and Physiology, The Sahlgrenska Academy at University of Gothenburg, Mölndal Campus, Mölndal, Sweden

JESSICA CHEW, BS
Ahmanson Translational Imaging Division, Department of Molecular and Medical Pharmacology, David Geffen School of Medicine at University of California, Los Angeles, California

JEFFREY L. CUMMINGS, MD, ScD
Director, Lou Ruvo Center for Brain Health in Las Vegas, Andrea and Joseph Hahn Chair of Neurological Institute, Cleveland Clinic, Las Vegas, Nevada

BRUNO DUBOIS, MD
Fédération de Neurologie, Hôpital de la Salpêtrière, Paris, France

FRANCESCO G. GARACI, PhD
Associate Professor in Radiology, Department of Diagnostic Imaging and Interventional Radiology, University of Rome "Tor Vergata"; IRCCS San Raffaele Pisana, Roma, Italy

MICHEL GROTHE, PhD
DZNE, German Center for Neurodegenerative Diseases, Rostock, Germany

HARALD HAMPEL, MD
Department of Psychiatry, Goethe University, Frankfurt, Germany

JOHN HARRISON, CSci, CPsychol, PhD
Honorary Senior Lecturer, Department of Medicine, Imperial College, London, United Kingdom; Principal Consultant, Metis Cognition Ltd, Wiltshire, United Kingdom

SIMONE LISTA, PhD
Department of Psychiatry, Goethe University, Frankfurt, Germany

JOSÉ L. MOLINUEVO, MD, PhD
Neurology Service, Alzheimer's Disease and Other Cognitive Disorders Unit, Hospital Clínic; Institut d'Investigació Biomédica August Pi I Sunyer (Neurodegenerative Diseases Group); ICN Hospital Clinic i Universitari and Pasqual Maragall Foundation, Barcelona, Spain

FLORENCE PASQUIER, MD, PhD
Professor, University Lille Nord de France; UDSL, EA1046, CHU de Lille, Lille, France; Department of Neurology, Memory Center, University Lille 2, CHRU, Lille Cedex, France

JAGAN A. PILLAI, MBBS, PhD
Lou Ruvo Center for Brain Health, Cleveland Clinic, Cleveland, Ohio

LORENA RAMI, PhD
Neurology Service, Alzheimer's Disease and Other Cognitive Disorders Unit, Hospital Clínic, Barcelona, Spain; Institut d'Investigació Biomédica August Pi i Sunyer (IDIBAPS), Spain

CHRISTOPHER C. ROWE, MD
Department of Nuclear Medicine, Centre for PET; Department of Medicine, University of Melbourne, Austin Health, Heidelberg, Victoria, Australia

PHILIP SCHELTENS, MD
Professor of Cognitive Neurology, Director of the Alzheimer Center, VU University Medical Center, Amsterdam, Netherlands

DANIEL H.S. SILVERMAN, MD, PhD
Head, Neuronuclear Imaging Section, Ahmanson Translational Imaging Division, Professor, Molecular and Medical Pharmacology, David Geffen School of Medicine at University of California, Los Angeles, California

STEFAN J. TEIPEL, MD
University Medicine Rostock; DZNE, German Center for Neurodegenerative Diseases, Rostock, Germany

NICOLA TOSCHI, PhD
Assistant Professor, Medical Physics Section, Faculty of Medicine, University of Rome "Tor Vergata", Rome, Italy

VICTOR L. VILLEMAGNE, MD
Department of Nuclear Medicine, Centre for PET; Department of Medicine, University of Melbourne, Austin Health, Heidelberg, Victoria, Australia

HENRIK ZETTERBERG, MD, PhD
Clinical Neurochemistry Laboratory, Institute of Neuroscience and Physiology, The Sahlgrenska Academy at University of Gothenburg, Mölndal Campus, Mölndal, Sweden

Contents

Magnetic resonance imaging (MRI)-based indicators of regional and global brain atrophy and more advanced measures of cortical functional and structural connectivity are among the most promising imaging biomarkers for the characterization of preclinical and prodromal stages of Alzheimer disease (AD). This review presents the current status of available and evolving MRI-based technologies for the early asymptomatic and predementia diagnosis of AD, including high-resolution structural MRI of global and regional brain atrophy, diffusion tensor imaging of structural cortical connectivity, and functional MRI during rest and task performance. The selection of an appropriate technique needs to consider its suitability for specific applications.

In this article, cognitive measures in the screening of individuals at risk for Alzheimer disease (AD) are reviewed. Use of cognitive tasks in identifying clinical cases of AD is considered, as well as methods for detecting those in the prodromal stages of the disease, including cognitive screening instruments. Traditional assessments, such as the mini-mental state examination, as well as contemporary computerized screening instruments, are examined. Areas of cognition for investigation in the detection of prodromal AD are recommended. The prospects for general cognitive screening are reviewed, and more engaging technologies to tests individuals at risk for developing AD are recommended.

Effective treatments of Alzheimer disease (AD) dementia are an urgent necessity. There is a growing consensus that effective disease-modifying treatment before the onset of clinical dementia and slowing the progression of mild symptoms are needed after recent setbacks in AD therapeutics. The identification of at-risk and preclinical AD populations is becoming important for targeting primary and secondary prevention clinical trials in AD. This article reviews the strategies and challenges in targeting at-risk and preclinical AD populations for a new generation of AD clinical trials. Design, outcome measures, and complexities in successfully completing a clinical trial targeting this population are reviewed.

This article reviews the current recommendations in early diagnosis and the desires of the patients and their relatives, put in perspective with the reality of the clinical practices. More specific situations covered are: (1) the issue of young diseased patients, taking into account the psychological implications of the early occurrence of the disease in life and of the longer delay for these patients between the first observable signs and the diagnosis and (2) the issue of genetic testing, taking into account the implications of this extremely early form of bad news on the individual's existence and on the family structure.

In 2007, new International Working Group research criteria introduced a new conceptualization of Alzheimer disease and created a framework for earlier diagnosis. There is increasing consensus to understand Alzheimer disease as a clinical-biologic entity, in which biomarkers, especially pathophysiologic markers revealing underlying pathology, represent the biologic counterpart of the diagnosis, and specific symptoms, such as episodic memory deficits, account for the clinical one. This article advances and moves forward on this.

^{18}F-fludeoxyglucose positron emission tomography (FDG-PET) is an important tool for detecting the early stages of Alzheimer disease (AD). This article discusses the multiple roles FDG-PET plays in helping to diagnose AD, including detecting the disease in the prodromal and early dementia stages, differential diagnosis of dementia, documenting and quantifying cognitive decline, and predicting progression from mild cognitive impairment to AD. In addition, the role of structural magnetic resonance imaging, underutilization of FDG-PET, and a suggested multimodal approach for early AD diagnosis are discussed.

Preface

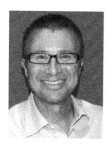 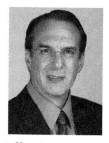 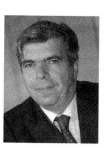 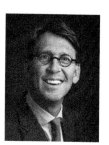

José L. Molinuevo,   Jeffrey L. Cummings,   Bruno Dubois, MD   Philip Scheltens, MD
MD, PhD   MD, ScD

Editors

Alzheimer disease (AD) has until recently been regarded as a dementia syndrome and diagnosis was not made until the patient evidenced sufficient cognitive decline to manifest a dementia syndrome with cognitive and functional decline. Definite diagnosis of AD required a postmortem confirmation. This conceptualization and diagnosis of AD are currently undergoing a major transformation, due to both the introduction of biomarkers into the field and the recognition that the clinical stage of the disease is preceded by a long silent asymptomatic phase and a predementia symptomatic period. The first meaningful step leading to this reconceptualization was taken by an International Working Group (IWG) led by Bruno Dubois in 2007. The IWG criteria offered a redefinition of AD as a dual clinicobiological entity that could be recognized in vivo, before the onset of dementia, on the basis of a specific core clinical phenotype comprised of an amnestic syndrome of the hippocampal type and supportive evidence from biomarkers reflecting the presence of an Alzheimer-type pathologic condition. A direct consequence of the introduction of the IWG criteria has been a redefinition of the disease—considered to be a clinicobiological entity—with a long asymptomatic period, the preclinical or presymptomatic stage, preceding the symptomatic one or clinical stage of the disease.

This shift in the conceptualization and diagnosis of AD opened the door for earlier and more specific, biomarker-supported, diagnosis of the disease. The diagnosis can now be established in the prodromal stage of the disease before the occurrence of dementia. This fact has already generated several consequences: initiation of clinical trials at a predementia stage with disease-modifying drugs and implementation in research and academic centers, earlier disease diagnosis, and investigation of early transitional stages of the disease from normal to mild impairment and from mild impairment to mild dementia. The clinical stage can now be detected in mildly symptomatic patients before dementia appears, offering the subject the possibility of making valuable decisions while still competent. Because there is consensus that the diagnosis should be implemented only in the clinical stage of the disease, the

Med Clin N Am 97 (2013) xiii–xv
http://dx.doi.org/10.1016/j.mcna.2013.01.003
0025-7125/13/$ – see front matter © 2013 Published by Elsevier Inc.

medical.theclinics.com

essence of the new IWG diagnostic criteria relies on the recognition of this dual aspect for the diagnosis of AD: a specific clinical presentation that is related to a well-defined underlying pathologic abnormality detected through biomarkers.

Biomarkers are required for the diagnosis of AD in the IWG approach. Patients must exhibit either pathophysiologic or topographic abnormalities characteristic of AD. Pathophysiologic markers include the molecular signature of AD in the cerebrospinal fluid of low amyloid beta (Aβ) peptide with elevated levels of tau or hyperphosphorylated tau or abnormal amyloid imaging with one of the available ligands specific for fibrillar Aβ. Topographic markers include medial temporal/hippocampal atrophy on magnetic resonance imaging or bilateral parietal hypometabolism on positron emission tomography. The increasing knowledge of biomarkers, their role in diagnosis and in determining disease evolution, and better understanding on the disease continuum, with its initial clinically silent preclinical stage and mildly symptomatic prodromal one, have completely shifted the AD field from the old conceptualization of AD as a dementia—not now recognized as the end-stage disease—into a highly evolving field of knowledge and potential early diagnoses and treatments. This volume presents a comprehensive view of this new understanding of the disease with the attendant possibilities offered by the biomarkers (both those currently in use and those being developed) as well as potential therapeutics.

This milestone volume shares the current, up-to-date knowledge and understanding of the possibilities offered not only by biomarkers but also by this new conceptualization of the disease. Each article, written by world-renowned experts, summarizes an area of knowledge relevant to early diagnosis and offers a window into the future on research and clinical practice. The issue also covers the state of the art on clinical trials for prodromal and very early AD and how the clinical diagnosis may evolve in the near future.

In summary, there is increasing consensus on AD as a clinicobiological entity in which biomarkers, especially pathophysiologic markers revealing the underlying pathologic condition, and clinical assessment reveal the corresponding clinical deficits. This reconceptualization of the disease is for the first time creating the possibility of intervening through clinical trials in the predementia stage of the disease. This issue crystalizes the current understanding and knowledge of AD by offering a thorough overview of the state of the art of this fascinating and evolving field.

José L. Molinuevo, MD, PhD
Neurology Service
Alzheimer's disease and other cognitive disorders unit
ICN Hospital Clinic i Universitari
and Pasqual Maragall Foundation
Barcelona, Spain

Jeffrey L. Cummings, MD, ScD
Lou Ruvo Center for Brain Health in Las Vegas
Cleveland Clinic
Las Vegas, NV, USA

Bruno Dubois, MD
Fédération de Neurologie
Hôpital de la Salpêtrière
Paris, France

Philip Scheltens, MD
Cognitive Neurology
Alzheimer Center
VU University Medical Center
Amsterdam, Netherlands

E-mail addresses:
JLMOLI@clinic.ub.es (J.L. Molinuevo)
cumminj@ccf.org (J.L. Cummings)
bruno.dubois@psl.aphp.fr (B. Dubois)
p.scheltens@vumc.nl (P. Scheltens)

International Work Group Criteria for the Diagnosis of Alzheimer Disease

Jeffrey L. Cummings, MD, ScD[a],*, Bruno Dubois, MD[b],
José L. Molinuevo, MD, PhD[d], Philip Scheltens, MD[c]

KEYWORDS

- International Work Group • Alzheimer disease • Diagnosis • Biomarkers

KEY POINTS

- Alzheimer-type biomarker changes are identifiable in asymptomatic and mildly symptomatic predementia phases of Alzheimer disease (AD) as well as AD dementia.
- The International Work Group (IWG) guidelines for diagnosis identify a unified spectrum of 3 phases, from at-risk state asymptomatic to symptomatic prodromal AD and AD dementia.
- The classic clinical feature that indicates AD is an episodic memory defect of the amnestic type; this is the key clinical aspect of prodromal AD and AD dementia.
- IWG criteria require biomarker support for the diagnosis of AD at any clinical stage.
- These criteria are proposed to allow highly specific diagnosis of AD and assist in identifying patients for clinical trials of AD-related treatments and other types of AD research.

Disclosure: JLM has provided scientific advice or has been an investigator or data monitoring board member for consultancy fees from Pfizer, Eisai, MSD, Merz, Janssen-Cilag, Novartis, Lundbeck, Roche, Bayer, Bristol-Myers Squibb, GE Health Care, GlaxoSmithKline, and Innogenetics. PS has provided scientific advice or has been an investigator or data monitoring board member for consultancy fees from Pfizer, Eisai, Merck, Genentech, Nutricia, Janssen AI, Novartis, Lundbeck, Roche, Bristol-Myers Squibb, GE Health Care, and Avid-Lilly. JLC has provided consultation for Abbott, Acadia, ADAMAS, Anavex, Astellas, Avanir, Baxter, Bristol-Myers Squibb, Eisai, Elan, EnVivo, Forest, Genentech, GlaxoSmithKline, Janssen, Lilly, Lundbeck, Medtronics, Merck, Neurokos, Neuronix, Novartis, Otsuka, Pain Therapeutics, Pfizer, Plexxicon, Prana, QR, Sanofi, Sonexa, Takeda, and Toyama pharmaceutical companies. JLC has provided consultation for assessment to the following companies: Bayer, Avid, GE, MedAvante, Neurotrax, and UBC. JLC owns stock in ADAMAS, Prana, Sonexa, MedAvante, Neurotrax, Neurokos, and QR pharma. JLC has been a speaker or lecturer for Eisai, Forest, Janssen, Novartis, Pfizer, Lundbeck. JLC owns the copyright of the Neuropsychiatric Inventory. JLC has provided expert witness consultation regarding olanzapine and ropinerol.
[a] Cleveland Clinic Lou Ruvo Center for Brain Health, 888 West Bonneville Avenue, Las Vegas, NV, USA; [b] Cleveland Clinic Lou Ruvo Center for Brain Health, Cleveland, OH, USA; [c] Alzheimer's Disease and Other Cognitive Disorders Unit, Hospital Clínic, Fundació Pasqual Maragall, Barcelona, Spain; [d] Department of Neurology, Alzheimer Center, VU University Medical Center, Amsterdam, The Netherlands
* Corresponding author. Cleveland Clinic Lou Ruvo Center for Brain Health, 888 West Bonneville Avenue, Las Vegas, NV 89106.
E-mail address: cumminj@ccf.org

Med Clin N Am 97 (2013) 363–368
http://dx.doi.org/10.1016/j.mcna.2013.01.001
0025-7125/13/$ – see front matter © 2013 Published by Elsevier Inc.

medical.theclinics.com

Alzheimer disease (AD) was defined as a type of dementia with the publication of the *National Institute of Neurologic and Communicative Disorders and Stroke–Alzheimer's Disease and Related Disorders* criteria in 1984.[1] Two major tenets of these criteria were that: (1) the diagnosis of AD could be made only when the disease is advanced and reaches the threshold of dementia; (2) even at this stage, the diagnosis of AD could only be probable, because diagnostic certainty requires postmortem confirmation. In 2007, an International Work Group (IWG) led by Bruno Dubois offered a redefinition of AD as a dual clinicobiological syndrome that can be recognized in vivo, before the onset of dementia, by (1) a specific core clinical phenotype comprising an amnestic syndrome of the hippocampal type and (2) supportive evidence from biomarkers reflecting the presence of Alzheimer-type pathology using IWG criteria. AD is diagnosed with the same criteria throughout all symptomatic phases of the disease (IWG/Dubois criteria).[2] The definitions were further clarified in 2010.[3] The major advance of the IWG criteria was to integrate the use of biomarkers into diagnosis to allow a biologically based approach to diagnosis integrated with clinical manifestations but independent of disease severity. A key point is that AD occurs along a spectrum of severity, and criteria that reflect the seamless progression of symptoms from the mildest to the most severe forms of the disease are needed.

IWG CRITERIA FOR THE DIAGNOSIS OF AD

Box 1 provides the current version of the IWG criteria for the diagnosis of AD. The clinical syndrome is the critical aspect of the diagnosis. Patients typically show an amnestic type of memory defect of the hippocampal type. Memory abnormalities should have been present for at least 6 months and should be documented by appropriate neuropsychological tests. The Free and Cued Selective Reminding Test has been shown to predict the presence of AD pathology in the hippocampus and is recommended as a means of capturing the typical clinical abnormality of AD.[4] Atypical forms of the disease are recognized and include posterior cortical, aphasic, and frontal types of presentations.

Biomarkers are required for the diagnosis of AD in the IWG approach. Patients must show either pathophysiologic or topographic abnormalities characteristic of AD. Pathophysiologic markers include the molecular signature of AD in the cerebrospinal fluid (CSF) of low amyloid β (Aβ) peptide plus increased levels of tau or hyperphosphorylated tau (p-tau) or abnormal amyloid imaging with one of the available ligands specific for fibrillar Aβ. Topographic markers include medial temporal/hippocampal atrophy or magnetic resonance imaging (MRI) or bilateral parietal hypometabolism on positron emission tomography.

Several phases of AD are recognized by the IWG criteria. Patients who have no symptoms but show the biomarkers of AD are recognized to be in an AD risk state. Approximately 20% to 30% of individuals older than 70 years have reduced $A\beta_{1-42}$ protein in the CSF and deposits of fibrillar Aβ in the brain that can be visualized by amyloid imaging.[5,6] Progression to AD is a high risk but it is unknown if all patients progress. Some patients succumb from competitive mortality of the elderly before manifesting clinical aspects of the disease and never have AD, despite a positive biomarker. Others might never progress within an expected life span. For this reason, we avoid the use of the term Alzheimer disease for this state, preferring to preserve the use of the term disease for those who have symptoms.

One rare exception to the statement that progression from the asymptomatic to the symptomatic state is unknown involves patients who have autosomal-dominant mutations causative of AD. Patients with presenilin 1 or amyloid precursor protein

---

Box 1
IWG criteria for the diagnosis of AD

Probable AD: A plus 1 or more supportive features B, C, D, or E

Core diagnostics criteria

A. Presence of an early and significant episodic memory impairment that includes the following features:

    a. Gradual and progressive change in memory function over more than 6 months

    b. Objective evidence of significantly impaired episodic memory consists of recall deficit that does not improve significantly with cueing or recognition testing and after effective encoding of information

    c. The episodic memory impairment can be isolated or associated with other cognitive changes at the onset of AD or as AD advances to dementia

Supportive features

B. Presence of medial temporal lobe atrophy

    a. Volume loss of hippocampi, entorhinal cortex, amygdala shown on MRI

C. Abnormal cerebrospinal fluid biomarker

    a. Low amyloid β_{1-42} concentrations, increased total tau or p-tau concentrations

    b. Other well-validated markers to be discovered in the future

D. Specific pattern on functional neuroimaging with positron emission tomography

    a. Reduced glucose metabolism in bilateral temporal-parietal regions

    b. Other well-validated ligands, including amyloid imaging

E. Proven AD autosomal-dominant mutation

Data from Dubois B, Feldman HH, Jacova C, et al. Research criteria for the diagnosis of Alzheimer's disease: revising the NINCDS-ADRDA criteria [review]. Lancet Neurol 2007; 6(8):734–46; and Dubois B, Feldman HH, Jacova C, et al. Revising the definition of Alzheimer's disease: a new lexicon. Lancet Neurol 2010;9(11):1118–27.

---

mutations universally progress to early-onset dementia and most patients with presenilin 2 mutations also have this fate. Given the high certainty of progression to early-onset symptomatic AD, the IWG recognizes this group as having preclinical AD.

Prodromal AD is the syndrome characterized by an amnestic type of memory impairment or one of the known atypical presentations of AD, a molecular biomarker that indicates AD, as described earlier, and no impairment of activities of daily living (ADLs). The preservation of ADLs indicates that the disability associated with AD has not progressed sufficiently to warrant the diagnosis of AD dementia. The diagnosis of prodromal AD differs from the nonspecific syndrome of mild cognitive impairment (MCI) in requiring a more specific clinical syndrome and having a biomarker that indicates AD. MCI is a heterogeneous disorder with outcomes that vary from recovery, to remaining in the MCI state, to progression to AD, to progression to non-AD types of dementia.[7] The IWG requirement for the biomarker of AD for prodromal AD increases the specificity of diagnosis and predicts progression over time to AD dementia.

AD dementia shows a memory impairment of the hippocampal type, has the molecular signature of AD, and entails impaired ADLs. The requirement for impaired ADLs distinguishes AD dementia from prodromal AD and establishes a continuum between the 2 syndromes distinguished only by the ADL aspect. All other requirements for the diagnosis of symptomatic AD are the same for prodromal AD and AD dementia, although in most cases, the cognitive deficits of AD dementia are more severe and involve a broader array of cognitive deficits (**Box 1**).

ADVANTAGES OF THE IWG CRITERIA

There are 3 major strengths of the IWG/Dubois criteria. First, they identify a clinicobiological syndrome using cognitive assessment and biomarker evidence that provides a framework for diagnosis of AD throughout any phase of AD after the onset of symptoms. The combination of a specific phenotype episodic memory impairment) and a biomarker supportive of the presence of Alzheimer pathology is the basis for diagnosis of AD at any stage of the disease.

Second, the IWG/Dubois criteria require the presence of a positive biomarker to diagnose AD, for any stage of the disease. This strategy takes advantage of recent rapid advances in our understanding of the biology of AD and the ability to identify the presence of AD pathology in vivo. Without this progress, there would be no need for new diagnostic criteria. The new diagnostic criteria and their application to earlier forms of disease are based on our emerging ability to use biomarkers to detect the earliest changes of the disease state before dementia supervenes. Amyloid abnormalities have been shown to be the earliest detectable changes in the biology of AD, to remain largely stable after the initial phases of the illness, and to correlate only weakly if at all with clinical measures.[8,9] Neurodegeneration biomarkers, including atrophy on MRI and increased CSF tau and p-tau are believed to begin later in AD, progress throughout the course of the disease, and correlate with indices of progressive clinical decline.[10–13]

Third, the IWG/Dubois criteria, by using a standard diagnostic approach with integrated biomarkers, identify a total of 4 diagnostic groups: asymptomatic at-risk state individuals with positive biomarkers; preclinical AD with an autosomal-dominant mutation; prodromal AD with episodic memory loss and a biomarker for AD; and AD dementia (**Table 1**). This modest complexity facilitates uniform application of the criteria in clinical and research settings.

The IWG/Dubois criteria embrace the entire continuum of symptomatic AD from the prodromal to the dementia forms in a single diagnostic framework; integrate biomarkers into all phases of the diagnostic approach; use biomarkers to improve on the diagnostic specificity of less specific syndromes such as MCI and AD dementia; emphasize episodic memory impairment as the key AD phenotype; and have the advantage of simplicity of application. Conceptually, they advance the idea of AD as a clinicobiological entity.

IWG/Dubois criteria for prodromal AD have been successfully implemented in clinical trials approved by the US Food and Drug Administration, and they have been accepted by the European Medicine Agency[13] for use in AD clinical trials.

Table 1		
Diagnosis recognized by the IWG criteria		
Disorder	**Clinical Manifestations**	**Biomarker Required**
AD risk state	None	Biomarker consistent with AD
Preclinical AD	None	Autosomal-dominant mutation causative of AD
Prodromal AD	Episodic memory loss or recognized atypical presentation; preserved ADL	Biomarker consistent with AD
AD dementia	Episodic memory loss or recognized atypical presentation; impaired ADL	Biomarker consistent with AD

IMPLICATIONS OF THE PREDEMENTIA DIAGNOSIS OF AD

Knowledge of the biology of AD and particularly the earliest changes of the disease is rapidly growing. Biomarker information allows the recognition of AD-type abnormalities before the onset of dementia and, in some cases, before the onset of any cognitive changes. The recognition of prodromal/predementia AD allows appreciation of the true sociobiological magnitude of the problem of AD. AD is at least twice as common as previous estimates of AD dementia suggest and is present in the brains of approximately 65% of 80-year olds.[8,9] Unless means of prevention and treatment are found, AD will afflict approximately 200,000,000 individuals by the year 2050, twice previous estimates based on the more advanced state of AD dementia.[14]

Earlier diagnosis means that the individuals live with the diagnosis longer, with profound effects on clinical care, caregiver support, and resource use. The psychological and emotional ramifications of early diagnosis without adequate therapy require thorough consideration from the scientific and care communities and society.[15] On the other hand, an early diagnosis allows life planning, decision making, clinical trial participation, and treatment when therapies become available.

NEXT STEPS

The IWG/Dubois criteria aim to capitalize on the emerging opportunity to integrate molecular biomarkers of Alzheimer pathology into a diagnostic framework for earlier clinical diagnosis. Use of biomarkers in research assists with clinical trials and possibly with regulatory decisions. They set the stage for primary prevention. The emphasis on biomarkers builds on an increasingly robust scientific basis, but data are emerging, and verification of the type of changes, correlations with clinical outcomes, order of appearance, and consistency across populations is required.

Criteria for the diagnosis of AD will benefit from validation studies and further investigation of their sensitivity, specificity, positive and negative predictive value, and clinical usefulness. Criteria might be improved by incorporating the emerging genetic information such as apolipoprotein E genotype. New biomarkers and possibly treatment responses in subgroups of AD may play a role in future evolutions of the diagnostic criteria.

REFERENCES

1. McKhann G, Drachman D, Folstein M, et al. Clinical diagnosis of Alzheimer's disease: report of the NINCDS-ADRDA Work Group under the auspices of Department of Health and Human Services Task Force on Alzheimer's Disease. Neurology 1984;34(7):939–44.
2. Dubois B, Feldman HH, Jacova C, et al. Research criteria for the diagnosis of Alzheimer's disease: revising the NINCDS-ADRDA criteria [review]. Lancet Neurol 2007;6(8):734–46.
3. Dubois B, Feldman HH, Jacova C, et al. Revising the definition of Alzheimer's disease: a new lexicon. Lancet Neurol 2010;9(11):1118–27.
4. Sarazin M, Berr C, De Rotrou J, et al. Amnestic syndrome of the medial temporal type identifies prodromal AD: a longitudinal study. Neurology 2007;69(19):1859–67.
5. Aizenstein HJ, Nebes RD, Saxton JA, et al. Frequent amyloid deposition without significant cognitive impairment among the elderly. Arch Neurol 2008;65(11):1509–17.
6. Villemagne VL, Rowe CC. Amyloid imaging. Int Psychogeriatr 2011;23:S41–9.

7. Jicha GA, Parisi JE, Dickson DW, et al. Neuropathologic outcome of mild cognitive impairment following progression to clinical dementia. Arch Neurol 2006; 63(5):674–81.

8. Villemagne VL, Pike KE, Chételat G, et al. Longitudinal assessment of Aβ and cognition in aging and Alzheimer disease. Ann Neurol 2011;69(1):181–92.

9. Rowe CC, Ellis KA, Rimajova M, et al. Amyloid imaging results from the Australian Imaging, Biomarkers and Lifestyle (AIBL) study of aging. Neurobiol Aging 2010; 31(8):1275–83.

10. Lo RY, Hubbard AE, Shaw LM, et al, for the Alzheimer's Disease Neuroimaging Initiative. Longitudinal change of biomarkers in cognitive decline. Arch Neurol 2011;68:1257–66.

11. Eckerstrom C, Andreasson U, Olsson E, et al. Combination of hippocampal volume and cerebrospinal fluid biomarkers improves predictive value in mild cognitive impairment. Dement Geriatr Cogn Disord 2010;29(4):294–300.

12. Jack CR Jr, Knopman DS, Jagust WJ, et al. Hypothetical model of dynamic biomarkers of the Alzheimer's pathological cascade. Lancet Neurol 2010;9(1): 119–28.

13. Isaac M, Vamvakas S, Abadie E, et al. Qualification opinion of novel methodologies in the predementia stage of Alzheimer's disease: cerebrospinal fluid related biomarkers for drug affecting amyloid burden–regulatory considerations by European Medicines Agency focusing in improving benefit/risks in regulatory trials. Eur Neuropsychopharmacol 2011;21:781–8.

14. Alzheimer's Association, Thies W, Bleiler L. 2011 Alzheimer's disease facts and figures. Alzheimers Dement 2011;7(2):208–44.

15. Karlawish J. Addressing the ethical, policy and social challenges of preclinical Alzheimer's disease. Neurology 2011;77:1487–93.

The Application of Cerebrospinal Fluid Biomarkers in Early Diagnosis of Alzheimer Disease

Kaj Blennow, MD, PhD*, Henrik Zetterberg, MD, PhD

KEYWORDS

- Alzheimer disease • Cerebrospinal fluid • Biomarkers • Early diagnosis
- Amyloid of Aβ • Tau protein

KEY POINTS

- Alzheimer disease (AD) dementia represents an advanced stage of the disease, with severe neuropathology with not only abundant plaque and tangle disease but also a marked synaptic and neuronal degeneration and loss.
- Research progress during the last 2 decades has resulted in brain imaging, in particular magnetic resonance imaging (MRI) and positron emission tomography (PET), and cerebrospinal fluid biomarkers that facilitate an accurate diagnosis of AD already during the mild cognitive impairment stage.
- Brain imaging biomarkers include MRI measurements of hippocampal volume to gauge brain atrophy, as well as PET measurements of [18F]fluorodeoxyglucose to assess glucose metabolism rate in brain cells (neurons and glial cells) in specific brain regions, as well as global cortical retention of amyloid binding ligands such as Pittsburgh Compound B.
- The CSF biomarkers Aβ42, total tau and phosphorylated tau show high diagnostic accuracy for AD also in the early clinical phases of the disease.
- Longitudinal clinical biomarker studies with multiple assessments will provide information on the temporal evolution of pathogenic mechanisms in the disease.

INTRODUCTION

The clinical criteria by the Neurologic and Communicative Disorders and Stroke and the Alzheimer's Disease and Related Disorders Association for diagnosing Alzheimer disease (AD) with dementia was outlined more than 25 years ago, at a time when there was no therapy available for the disease.[1] The launch of cholinesterase inhibitors for symptomatic treatment (for review see Ref.[2]) highlighted the importance of accurate diagnosis of AD with dementia.

Clinical Neurochemistry Laboratory, Institute of Neuroscience and Physiology, The Sahlgrenska Academy at University of Gothenburg, Mölndal Campus, Mölndal SE-43180, Sweden
* Corresponding author. Clinical Neurochemistry Laboratory, Institute of Neuroscience and Physiology, Sahlgrenska University Hospital, The Sahlgrenska Academy at University of Gothenburg, Mölndal Campus, Mölndal SE-43180, Sweden.
E-mail address: kaj.blennow@neuro.gu.se

Med Clin N Am 97 (2013) 369–376
http://dx.doi.org/10.1016/j.mcna.2012.12.012
0025-7125/13/$ – see front matter © 2013 Elsevier Inc. All rights reserved.

However, it has become evident that AD dementia represents an advanced stage of the disease, with severe neuropathology with not only abundant plaque and tangle disease but also a marked synaptic and neuronal degeneration and loss. The increasing number of failed phase 2 and 3 trials on anti-Aβ disease-modifying drug candidates in patients with AD dementia also suggest that this type of treatment must be initiated before neurodegeneration is too widespread and severe.[3] For this reason, it is preferable to perform clinical trials in the mild cognitive impairment (MCI) stage of AD, with mild symptoms only in the form of disturbances of episodic memory.[4] However, MCI is not a disease, but a heterogeneous syndrome caused by many disorders other than AD. Testing new drugs in clinical trials on an unselected MCI cohort would mean that around half of the cases do not have underlying AD, the disorder for which the drug is intended, which would introduce too much noise to allow identifying any clinical effect of the drug.

This situation has created a need for biomarkers as diagnostic tools for the diagnosis of AD. Research progress during the last 2 decades has resulted in brain imaging, in particular magnetic resonance imaging (MRI) and positron emission tomography (PET), and cerebrospinal fluid (CSF) biomarkers that facilitate an accurate diagnosis of AD already during the MCI stage (for review see Ref.[5]). Accordingly, in 2007, Dubois and colleagues[6] presented novel research criteria for the diagnosis of prodromal AD (ie, before the dementia stage), which are based on a clinical core of early and significant episodic memory impairment together with at least 1 or more abnormal biomarkers of the following: structural neuroimaging with MRI, molecular neuroimaging with PET, and CSF analyses of amyloid β and tau protein.

Brain imaging biomarkers include MRI measurements of hippocampal volume to gauge brain atrophy, as well as PET measurements of [^{18}F]fluorodeoxyglucose (FDG) to assess glucose metabolism rate in brain cells (neurons and glial cells) in specific brain regions, as well as global cortical retention of amyloid binding ligands such as Pittsburgh compound B.[5] This review focuses on CSF biomarkers for AD and their application in early AD diagnosis.

CSF BIOMARKERS FOR AD

Because of its proximity to the brain parenchyma and the free exchange with the brain extracellular space, the biochemical composition of CSF provides information of the brain chemistry. In contrast, peripheral blood (serum and plasma) is separated from the brain by the blood-brain barrier, and the minute amounts of brain proteins that may enter the blood are also diluted in a compartment containing high levels of other proteins such as albumin and IgG, and subjected to degradation by proteases and clearance in the liver or kidneys, which limits the potential of blood samples as biomarker sources for AD.

The unique characteristics of CSF, together with the low incidence of complications after lumbar puncture (LP) and CSF sampling (only a few patients admitted for evaluation of cognitive disturbances undergoing LP experience mild headache)[7] have contributed to introducing LP and analyses of CSF biomarkers into routine clinical practice in many centers.[8,9]

VALIDATED CSF BIOMARKERS FOR AD

In 1993, a first publication reported increased CSF levels of total tau (T-tau) in patients with AD with dementia.[10] Two years later, in 1995, increased CSF levels of phosphorylated tau (P-tau)[11] and decreased concentrations of the 42 amino acid isoform of Aβ (Aβ42)[12] was reported. Since this report, these 3 CSF biomarkers for AD have been evaluated in numerous publications. The most commonly used analytical methods are enzyme-linked immunosorbent assay (ELISA) methods, including assays for T-tau that measure all tau isoforms irrespective of phosphorylation state,[11] for tau phosphorylated at threonine 181 (P-tau181),[13] and for Aβ 1-42.[14] In 2005, a method for simultaneous analysis of these biomarkers in the same aliquot of CSF was published.[15] Although absolute levels differ for the individual biomarkers, ELISA and Luminex values correlate tightly, and the techniques show comparable diagnostic accuracy.[15]

All clinical CSF studies have consistently found an increase in CSF T-tau to around 300% of the level in cognitively normal elderly individuals, and a less pronounced increase in CSF P-tau to around 200%, whereas CSF Aβ42 is reduced to approximately 50% the level in normal elderly individuals.[16] These CSF biomarkers are 80% to 95% sensitive and specific for AD in the dementia phase of the disease.[16,17] Combined analyses of the biomarkers give a better diagnostic performance than any of the biomarkers by itself.[18–20] The CSF level of these markers is within the normal range in many important differential diagnoses, including depression and Parkinson disease.[2,17] Further, measurement of P-tau in CSF gives substantial aid to differentiate AD from other dementias, such as frontotemporal dementia and Lewy body dementia, but there are only marginal differences between assays specific for various P-tau epitopes, such as P-tau181, P-tau231 and P-tau199.[21] The diagnostic performance of these CSF biomarkers has also been validated in studies in which the diagnosis subsequently was confirmed by autopsy,[22,23] with similar or better discriminatory power than in studies based on patients with clinical diagnoses only.

CSF BIOMARKERS IN PRODROMAL AD

To enable early diagnosis of AD, it would be valuable if biomarkers were positive already when the first clinical symptoms occur, in the MCI phase of the disease. In 1999, Andreasen and colleagues[24] showed that patients with MCI who progress to AD with dementia during clinical follow-up have decreased CSF Aβ42 together with increased T-tau and P-tau. CSF biomarker levels were stable at follow-up, and the degree of biomarker abnormality was similar to that found after conversion to dementia.[24]

In the first study with an extended clinical follow-up period, which is needed to be more certain that stable MCI does not progress, Hansson and colleagues[19] showed that AD-indicative biomarker patterns are not seen in patients with MCI who remain stable or progress to other dementias. In the study reported in this article, 54 of 57 (sensitivity 95%) of prodromal AD cases had positive CSF biomarkers, at a specificity of 92% against controls and 83% against stable MCI cases and patients with MCI with progression to other dementias.[19] A high diagnostic accuracy of CSF biomarkers for prodromal AD has also been verified in several large multicenter studies, including the US ADNI (US Alzheimer's Disease Neuroimaging Initative) study,[23] the European DESCRIPA (Development of Screening guidelines and Criteria for Predementia Alzheimer's disease) study,[25] and the Swedish Brain Power project.[20] These results show that CSF biomarkers can serve as valuable clinical diagnostic tools to identify MCI cases with prodromal AD.

CSF BIOMARKERS IN PRECLINICAL AD

In 2003, Skoog and colleagues[26] showed that cognitively normal 85-year-olds who later developed dementia had decreased CSF Aβ42, but normal T-tau and P-tau levels. This finding was later confirmed in a population-based cohort of healthy elderly individuals aged 70 to 78 years with 8-year follow-up[27] and a clinical study on asymptomatic elderly individuals aged 60 to 94 years.[28] These findings suggest that in the sporadic form of AD, the CSF level of Aβ42 starts to decrease during the preclinical phase, before any evident increases in T-tau or P-tau.

Findings are less clear in familial AD (FAD). In 2005, Moonis and colleagues[29] published an article on CSF biomarkers in FAD, showing that asymptomatic individuals carrying FAD mutations have low CSF Aβ42 and high T-tau. This finding was corroborated by Ringman and colleagues,[30] who showed that mutation carriers have the full AD pattern of CSF biomarker changes with low CSF Aβ42 and high T-tau and P-tau. A recent longitudinal study also suggested that CSF levels of Aβ42 start to decline already 25 years before the expected clinical onset in FAD mutation carriers, whereas increased CSF tau may be found 15 years before expected symptom onset.[31] Taken together, these findings suggest that also in FAD, CSF biomarkers, especially CSF Aβ42, convert to positive many years before the first clinical symptoms in AD appear. It has also been noted that FAD mutation carriers in their early 20s may start off at significantly higher CSF Aβ42 concentrations than nonmutation carriers.[31,32] Longitudinal studies with repeated CSF samplings are needed to determine when and how fast the switch to lower CSF Aβ42 levels, indicating onset of amyloid deposition, occurs.

THE TEMPORAL EVOLUTION OF BIOMARKERS FOR AD

Clinically oriented AD researchers have focused much attention on the hypothetical model for the sequence of pathologic events in AD proposed by Jack and colleagues.[33] According to this hypothesis, biomarkers reflecting Aβ disease become positive before those reflecting neuronal degeneration and tangle formation.[33]

Two studies during the last year[34,35] have addressed this issue specifically. Both studies examined MCI cohorts with long clinical follow-up, and found a marked decrease in CSF Aβ42 accompanied by increases in CSF T-tau and P-tau. Although the outcome was similar, the interpretation of results differed. One study[34] showed that patients with MCI with prodromal AD have low CSF Aβ42, regardless of time to dementia, whereas T-tau and P-tau were highest in patients with shorter time to conversion, suggesting that Aβ42 is fully changed before T-tau or P-tau. These results provide direct support in humans for the hypothesis that altered Aβ metabolism precedes tau-related disease and neuronal degeneration. Another study[35] showed that patients with MCI with high levels of injury markers (ie, T-tau and P-tau) may progress faster, and thus have shorter time to conversion.

Both of these studies were cross-sectional, with 1 LP taken at baseline and clinical follow-up. Studies with multiple longitudinal CSF samples are needed to identify the time point at which the CSF biomarkers change from normal to pathologic values. The outcome of such studies may be either that CSF Aβ42 is stable reduced during the whole MCI phase, whereas T-tau and P-tau increase the closer to dementia the patient comes, or alternatively that all of Aβ42, T-tau, and P-tau is changed, but stable, during the whole MCI phase, with T-tau and P-tau predicting time to conversion. The longest longitudinal study to date[36] found remarkably stable CSF biomarker levels in 3 longitudinal CSF samples over 4 years in patients with MCI.

IMPLEMENTING CSF BIOMARKERS IN THE CLINIC

As reviewed earlier, CSF biomarkers for AD have been evaluated in numerous publications, which consistently have shown a high diagnostic accuracy both for AD dementia and for prodromal AD. A flow chart is presented for how the specific AD biomarkers can be implemented in clinical evaluation of patients with mild memory problems or other cognitive symptoms, which also follows the recommendations in the Dubois criteria from 2007[6] for the diagnosis of prodromal AD (**Fig. 1**). In addition

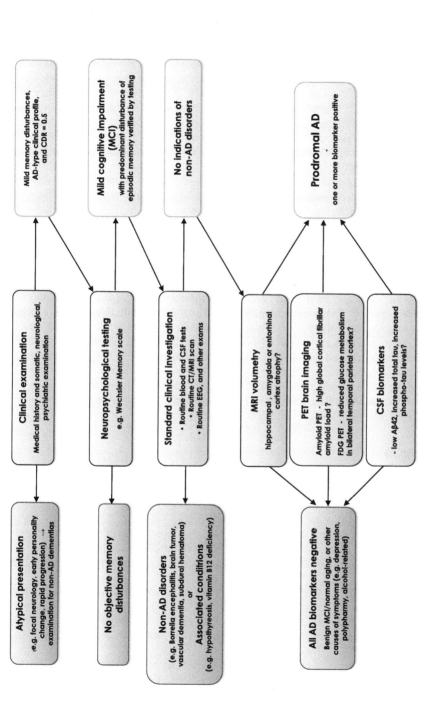

Fig. 1. Flow chart for implementing AD biomarkers in the examination of patients with mild memory problems and for diagnosis of prodromal AD.

to routine clinical diagnosis, CSF biomarkers are also increasingly used for enrichment of AD cases in many clinical trials.

However, although the CSF biomarkers assays show good performance in the monocenter setting,[8,9,37] there is a large variability in measurements between clinical centers and laboratories.[38] A flow chart with recommendations for standardization of preanalytical (LP and sample handling) procedures has been published.[2] However, there is also large between-laboratory variability, even when analyzing aliquots of the same sample,[38] which may be caused by differences in laboratory procedures (eg, pipetting, calibration of instruments and other equipment and postanalytical data handling), as well as variability in assay manufacturing leading to within-plate and between-plate variation and lot-to-lot variability (eg, calibrator purity and stability, coating of wells and antibody.[39]

This type of between-laboratory variability is by no means unique to CSF biomarkers, but is a general problem for all novel fluid biomarkers within clinical medicine. Several initiatives have been launched to develop certified reference materials to serve as gold standards for CSF biomarker measurements[39] and reference methods for analysis.[40] A candidate reference method for absolute quantification of $A\beta 1-38$, $A\beta 1-40$, and $A\beta 1-42$ that works on human CSF samples has recently been published.[41] A proficiency program for CSF biomarkers, the Alzheimer's Association Quality Control Program for CSF Biomarkers, has also been running for more than 2 years, with the aim to monitor between-laboratory and longitudinal variations in CSF biomarkers.[38] These programs, together with recent initiatives by the biotechnology industry to develop high-quality assays produced with rigorous quality-control measures that can run on fully automated instruments, will minimize variations and allow uniform cutoff levels for diagnosis and widespread use of CSF biomarkers in the clinical diagnostic setting and in clinical trials. Standardization efforts are also ongoing for other AD biomarkers, including MRI hippocampal volumetry.[42] The MRI standardization and assay validation process may also be valuable for other imaging biomarkers such as FDG and amyloid PET.[42]

REFERENCES

1. McKhann G, Drachman D, Folstein M, et al. Clinical diagnosis of Alzheimer's disease: report of the NINCDS-ADRDA Work Group under the auspices of Department of Health and Human Services Task Force on Alzheimer's Disease. Neurology 1984;34:939–44.
2. Blennow K, Hampel H, Weiner M, et al. Cerebrospinal fluid and plasma biomarkers in Alzheimer disease. Nat Rev Neurol 2010;6:131–44.
3. Blennow K. Biomarkers in Alzheimer's disease drug development. Nat Med 2010; 16:1218–22.
4. Petersen RC, Smith GE, Waring SC, et al. Mild cognitive impairment: clinical characterization and outcome. Arch Neurol 1999;56:303–8.
5. Hampel H, Frank R, Broich K, et al. Biomarkers for Alzheimer's disease: academic, industry and regulatory perspectives. Nat Rev Drug Discov 2010;9: 560–74.
6. Dubois B, Feldman HH, Jacova C, et al. Research criteria for the diagnosis of Alzheimer's disease: revising the NINCDS-ADRDA criteria. Lancet Neurol 2007; 6:734–46.
7. Zetterberg H, Tullhög K, Hansson O, et al. Low incidence of post-lumbar puncture headache in 1,089 consecutive memory clinic patients. Eur Neurol 2010; 63:326–30.

8. Andreasen N, Minthon L, Davidsson P, et al. Evaluation of CSF-tau and CSF-Aβ42 as diagnostic markers for Alzheimer's disease in clinical practice. Arch Neurol 2001;58:373–9.
9. Tabaraud F, Leman JP, Milor AM, et al. Alzheimer CSF biomarkers in routine clinical setting. Acta Neurol Scand 2012;125:416–23.
10. Vandermeeren M, Mercken M, Vanmechelen E, et al. Detection of tau proteins in normal and Alzheimer's disease cerebrospinal fluid with a sensitive sandwich enzyme-linked immunosorbent assay. J Neurochem 1993;61:1828–34.
11. Blennow K, Wallin A, Agren H, et al. Tau protein in cerebrospinal fluid: a biochemical marker for axonal degeneration in Alzheimer disease? Mol Chem Neuropathol 1995;26:231–45.
12. Motter R, Vigo-Pelfrey C, Kholodenko D, et al. Reduction of beta-amyloid peptide42 in the cerebrospinal fluid of patients with Alzheimer's disease. Ann Neurol 1995;38:643–8.
13. Vanmechelen E, Vanderstichele H, Davidsson P, et al. Quantification of tau phosphorylated at threonine 181 in human cerebrospinal fluid: a sandwich ELISA with a synthetic phosphopeptide for standardization. Neurosci Lett 2000;285:49–52.
14. Andreasen N, Hesse C, Davidsson P, et al. Cerebrospinal fluid β-amyloid(1-42) in Alzheimer's disease: differences between early- and late-onset Alzheimer disease and stability during the course of disease. Arch Neurol 1999;56:673–80.
15. Olsson A, Vanderstichele H, Andreasen N, et al. Simultaneous measurement of β-amyloid(1-42), tau and phosphorylated tau (Thr181) in cerebrospinal fluid by the xMAP technology. Clin Chem 2005;51:336–45.
16. Blennow K. Cerebrospinal fluid protein biomarkers for Alzheimer's disease. NeuroRx 2004;1:213–25.
17. Blennow K, Hampel H. Cerebrospinal fluid markers for incipient Alzheimer's disease. Lancet Neurol 2003;2:605–13.
18. Maddalena A, Papassotiropoulos A, Müller-Tillmanns B, et al. Biochemical diagnosis of Alzheimer disease by measuring the cerebrospinal fluid ratio of phosphorylated tau protein to beta-amyloid peptide42. Arch Neurol 2003;60:1202–6.
19. Hansson O, Zetterberg H, Buchhave P, et al. Association between CSF biomarkers and incipient Alzheimer's disease in patients with mild cognitive impairment: a follow-up study. Lancet Neurol 2006;5:228–34.
20. Mattsson N, Zetterberg H, Hansson O, et al. CSF biomarkers and incipient Alzheimer disease in patients with mild cognitive impairment. JAMA 2009;302:385–93.
21. Hampel H, Teipel SJ, Fuchsberger T, et al. Value of CSF β-amyloid1-42 and tau as predictors of Alzheimer's disease in patients with mild cognitive impairment. Mol Psychiatry 2004;9:705–10.
22. Koopman K, Le Bastard N, Martin JJ, et al. Improved discrimination of autopsy-confirmed Alzheimer's disease (AD) from non-AD dementias using CSF P-tau(181P). Neurochem Int 2009;55:214–8.
23. Shaw LM, Vanderstichele H, Knapik-Czajka M, et al, Alzheimer's Disease Neuroimaging Initiative. Cerebrospinal fluid biomarker signature in Alzheimer's disease neuroimaging initiative subjects. Ann Neurol 2009;65:403–13.
24. Andreasen N, Minthon L, Vanmechelen E, et al. CSF-tau and CSF-Aβ42 as predictors of development of Alzheimer's disease in patients with mild cognitive impairment. Neurosci Lett 1999;273:5–8.
25. Visser PJ, Verhey F, Knol DL, et al. Prevalence and prognostic value of cerebrospinal fluid markers of Alzheimer pathology in subjects with subjective cognitive impairment and mild cognitive impairment. The DESCRIPA study. Lancet Neurol 2009;8:619–27.

26. Skoog I, Davidsson P, Aevarsson O, et al. Cerebrospinal fluid beta-amyloid 42 is reduced before the onset of sporadic dementia: a population-based study in 85-year-olds. Dement Geriatr Cogn Disord 2003;15:169–76.

27. Gustafson DR, Skoog I, Rosengren L, et al. Cerebrospinal fluid β-amyloid 1-42 concentration may predict cognitive decline in older women. J Neurol Neurosurg Psychiatry 2007;78:461–4.

28. Stomrud E, Hansson O, Blennow K, et al. Cerebrospinal fluid biomarkers predict decline in subjective cognitive function over 3 years in healthy controls. Dement Geriatr Cogn Disord 2007;24:118–24.

29. Moonis M, Swearer JM, Dayaw MP, et al. Familial Alzheimer disease: decreases in CSF Abeta42 levels precede cognitive decline. Neurology 2005;65:323–5.

30. Ringman JM, Younkin SG, Pratico D, et al. Biochemical markers in persons with preclinical familial Alzheimer disease. Neurology 2008;71:85–92.

31. Bateman RJ, Xiong C, Benzinger TL, et al, Dominantly Inherited Alzheimer Network. Clinical and biomarker changes in dominantly inherited Alzheimer's disease. N Engl J Med 2012;367:795–804.

32. Reiman EM, Quiroz YT, Fleisher AS, et al. Brain imaging and fluid biomarker analysis in young adults at genetic risk for autosomal dominant Alzheimer's disease in the presenilin 1 E280A kindred: a case-control study. Lancet Neurol 2012;11(12):1048–56.

33. Jack CR Jr, Knopman DS, Jagust WJ, et al. Hypothetical model of dynamic biomarkers of the Alzheimer's pathological cascade. Lancet Neurol 2010;9:119–28.

34. Buchhave P, Minthon L, Zetterberg H, et al. Cerebrospinal fluid levels of β-amyloid 1-42, but not of tau, are fully changed already 5 to 10 years before the onset of Alzheimer's dementia. Arch Gen Psychiatry 2012;69:98–106.

35. van Rossum IA, Vos SJ, Burns L, et al. Injury markers predict cognitive decline in subjects with MCI and amyloid pathology. Neurology 2012;79:1809–16.

36. Mattsson N, Portelius E, Rolstad S, et al. Longitudinal cerebrospinal fluid biomarkers over four years in mild cognitive impairment. J Alzheimers Dis 2012;30:767–78.

37. Johansson P, Mattsson N, Hansson O, et al. Cerebrospinal fluid biomarkers for Alzheimer's disease: diagnostic performance in a homogeneous mono-center population. J Alzheimers Dis 2011;24:537–46.

38. Mattsson N, Andreasson U, Persson S, et al. The Alzheimer's Association external quality control program for CSF biomarkers. Alzheimers Dement 2011;7:386–95.

39. Mattsson N, Zegers I, Andreasson U, et al. Reference measurement procedures for Alzheimer's disease cerebrospinal fluid biomarkers: definitions and approaches with focus on amyloid β42. Biomark Med 2012;6:409–17.

40. Mattsson N, Andreasson U, Carrillo MC, et al. Proficiency testing programs for Alzheimer's disease cerebrospinal fluid biomarkers. Biomark Med 2012;6:401–7.

41. Pannee J, Portelius E, Oppermann M, et al. A selection reaction monitoring (SRM)-based method for absolute quantification of Aβ38, Aβ40 and Aβ42 in cerebrospinal fluid of Alzheimer disease patients and healthy controls. J Alzheimers Dis 2012;33:1021–32.

42. Jack CR Jr, Barkhof F, Bernstein MA, et al. Steps to standardization and validation of hippocampal volumetry as a biomarker in clinical trials and diagnostic criterion for Alzheimer's disease. Alzheimers Dement 2011;7:474–85.

Amyloid Imaging with PET in Early Alzheimer Disease Diagnosis

Christopher C. Rowe, MD[a,b,*], Victor L. Villemagne, MD[a,b]

KEYWORDS

- Alzheimer disease • Amyloid imaging • Posistron emission tomography • Aβ levels

KEY POINTS

- Amyloid imaging allows earlier diagnosis of Alzheimer disease (AD) and better differential diagnosis of dementia and provides prognostic information for individuals with mild cognitive impairment (MCI). It also has an increasingly important role in therapeutic trial recruitment and for the evaluation of anti-Aβ treatments.
- Many normal elderly people have elevated levels of Aβ and remain clinically normal for many years. It has been recently demonstrated that it takes up to 20 years for the Aβ burden to progress from an amount that is just detectable on positron emission tomography (PET) to that which is typical of patients with AD.
- Clear criteria for appropriate use are required and must emphasize the need to integrate the result of amyloid imaging with a comprehensive clinical and cognitive evaluation performed by clinicians experienced in the evaluation of dementia, to ensure a positive impact on patient management is achieved.

INTRODUCTION

AD is a progressive and irreversible neurodegenerative disorder clinically characterized by memory loss and cognitive decline that severely affect the activities of daily living.[1] AD is the leading cause of dementia in the elderly, leading invariably to death, usually within 7 to 10 years after diagnosis.[2] The progressive nature of the neurodegeneration suggests an age-dependent process that ultimately leads to synaptic failure and neuronal damage in cortical areas of the brain essential for memory and

This work was supported in part by grant 1011689 of the National Health and Medical Research Council of Australia, the Science and Industry Endowment Fund, and the Austin Hospital Medical Research Foundation.

[a] Department of Nuclear Medicine, Centre for PET, University of Melbourne, Austin Health, 145 Studley Road, Heidelberg, Victoria 3084, Australia; [b] Department of Medicine, University of Melbourne, Austin Health, 145 Studley Road, Heidelberg, Victoria 3084, Australia

* Corresponding author. Department of Nuclear Medicine and Centre for PET, University of Melbourne, Austin Health, 145 Studley Road, Heidelberg, Victoria 3084, Australia.
E-mail address: christopher.rowe@austin.org.au

other cognitive domains. AD not only has devastating effects on the sufferers and their caregivers but also has a tremendous socioeconomic impact on families and the health system; a burden that will only increase in the upcoming years as the population of most countries ages. In the absence of reliable biomarkers, direct pathologic examination of brain tissue derived from either biopsy or autopsy has been the only definitive method for establishing a diagnosis of AD. The typical macroscopic picture is gross cortical atrophy, whereas microscopically, there is widespread cellular degeneration and diffuse synaptic and neuronal loss, accompanied by reactive gliosis and the presence of the pathologic hallmarks of the disease: intracellular neurofibrillary tangles (NFTs) and extracellular amyloid plaques.[3,4] Although NFTs are intraneuronal bundles of paired helical filaments mainly composed of the aggregates of an abnormally phosphorylated form of tau protein,[5] neuritic plaques consist of dense extracellular aggregates of amyloid-β (Aβ),[6] surrounded by reactive gliosis and dystrophic neurites. Aβ is a 4-kDa 39–43 amino acid metalloprotein derived from the proteolytic cleavage of the amyloid precursor protein (APP), by β-secretases and γ-secretases.[7] To date, all available genetic, pathologic, biochemical, and cellular evidence strongly supports the notion that an imbalance between the production and removal of Aβ, leading to its progressive accumulation, is central to the pathogenesis of AD.[8] The Aβ-centric theory[1] postulates that Aβ plaque deposition is the primary event in a cascade of effects that lead to neurofibrillary degeneration and dementia.[9]

The clinical diagnosis of AD is still largely based on progressive impairment of memory and decline in at least one other cognitive domain and by excluding other diseases that might also present with dementia or pseudodementia, such as frontotemporal lobar degeneration (FTLD), dementia with Lewy bodies (DLB), stroke, brain tumor, normal pressure hydrocephalus, or depression. At this point, there is no cure for AD or proved way to slow the rate of neurodegeneration. Symptomatic treatment with an acetylcholinesterase inhibitor or a glutamatergic moderator provides modest benefit in some patients, usually by temporary stabilization rather than a noticeable improvement in memory function.

RECENT DEVELOPMENTS IN THE DIAGNOSIS OF ALZHEIMER DISEASE

The criteria for diagnosis of probable AD were described in 1984 and rely on establishing the presence of progressive impairment in memory and in at least one other area of cognition, such as language or visuoconstructional function, while excluding other causes. To meet these clinical criteria for AD, the cognitive impairment must be of sufficient severity to cause dementia (ie, prevent individuals from undertaking their usual occupation or daily activities).[10] Structural brain imaging with CT or MRI and blood screens have been recommended to exclude alternate causes of dementia, such as normal pressure hydrocephalus, hypothyroidism, and stroke. Clinical diagnosis compared with postmortem histopathologic diagnosis in most centers, however, is only 80% to 85% sensitive and 70% specific for AD.[11] Other causes of dementia, such as frontotemporal dementia and dementia with Lewy bodies, have many features in common with AD and are frequently misdiagnosed as AD. Recently, the diagnostic criteria for AD have been revisited and a new category created, termed *probable AD dementia with evidence of the AD pathophysiologic process*, by the 2011 National Institute on Aging and Alzheimer's Association workgroup.[12] This recommendation states that biomarkers (such as amyloid imaging) may be useful in 3 circumstances: in investigational studies, in clinical trials, and as optional clinical tools for use where available and when deemed appropriate by a clinician.

The most validated biomarkers for AD fall under 2 categories: (1) those that reflect the specific pathology of AD and (2) those that reflect neuronal damage or dysfunction. The pathology biomarkers of AD are Aβ imaging and cerebrospinal fluid (CSF) assay of the amyloid peptide, $A\beta_{42}$.[13] The pathology biomarkers are believed to be present before those biomarkers that reflect neuronal damage.[14] The biomarkers for neuronal damage or dysfunction are atrophy on MRI, parietotemporal hypometabolism on fluorodeoxyglucose (FDG)-PET, and elevation of CSF tau protein. In MRI, the location of atrophy adds specificity for AD and is most prominent in the hippocampi and adjacent entorhinal cortex.[15,16] In FDG-PET, the pattern of hypometabolism gives specificity for AD and is found in the lateral and medial (precuneus) posterior parietal, lateral temporal, and posterior cingulate cortex.[17] Tau and phosphorylated tau are released into CSF from damaged neurons, so although present in most cases of AD, they may be present for other reasons, including acute stroke. Aβ imaging shows increased tracer binding in cortical areas known to have high concentrations of amyloid plaques, in particular, the medial and orbitofrontal, lateral parietal and precuneus, lateral temporal, and posterior cingulate gyrus gray matter.[18,19]

A variable period of up to 5 years of prodromal decline in cognition characterized by an isolated impairment in short-term memory that may also be accompanied by impairments of working memory, known as amnestic MCI, usually precedes the formal diagnosis of AD.[20,21] Advances in biomarkers for AD have recently led to proposals for more definitive diagnoses in patients with MCI, such as prodromal AD, by the International Working Group for New Research Criteria for the Diagnosis of AD,[22] or mild cognitive impairment due to AD, by the National Institute on Aging and Alzheimer's Association workgroup[23]; recommendations by the latter define MCI due to AD as "high likelihood" when both an amyloid and a neurodegenerative biomarker are positive, as "intermediate likelihood" if just 1 biomarker is tested and is positive, or as MCI "unlikely due to AD" if both amyloid and neurodegenerative biomarkers are negative for AD. These diagnoses cannot be made on clinical grounds alone because patients with MCI proceed to other types of dementia in 10% to 20% of cases or prove not to have a progressive neurodegenerative condition on long-term follow-up in 30% to 40% of individuals.[20,24] Delaying diagnosis in a symptomatic person until dementia is apparent results in uncertainty and frustration for patients and their families; costly serial investigation; and delay in forward planning of employment, financial, and lifestyle options and future accommodation needs as well as delay in potentially beneficial symptomatic therapy. Alternatively, commencing therapy in MCI without other evidence to support the presence of prodromal AD leads to inappropriate medication use in the 50% of MCI patients who do not have AD. A potential future reason for earlier and more accurate diagnosis of AD is that disease-modifying therapies currently under development are more likely to be effective if given early, to slow or halt disease progression before extensive neuronal death and dementia has developed.

RADIOTRACERS FOR IMAGING BRAIN AMYLOID

PET is a sensitive molecular imaging technique that allows in vivo quantification of radiotracer concentrations in the picomolar range, allowing the noninvasive assessment of molecular processes at their sites of action, and is capable of detecting disease processes at asymptomatic stages when there is no evidence of anatomic change on MRI.[25] Because Aβ is at the center of AD pathogenesis, and given that several pharmacologic agents aimed at reducing Aβ levels in the brain are being developed and tested, many efforts have been focused on generating radiotracers for imaging Aβ in vivo.[26,27]

As a quantitative neuroimaging probe, the Aβ radiotracer must possess several key general properties: it should be a lipophilic, nontoxic small molecule with a high specificity and selectivity for Aβ and amenable for high specific activity labeling with fluorine-18 (^{18}F) or other long-lived radioisotopes, with no radiolabeled metabolites that enter the brain, while reversibly binding to Aβ in a specific and selective fashion.[28–30] Overall, binding affinity and lipophilicity are the most crucial properties for in vivo neuroimaging tracers. Although high affinity for Aβ is desirable to provide an adequate signal-to-noise ratio, this high affinity might also delay reaching binding equilibrium, requiring an extended scanning time. And although lipophilicity is necessary for the tracer to cross the blood-brain barrier, if the radiotracer is too lipophilic, its nonspecific binding might be too high.[28,30]

Through the years, several compounds have been evaluated as potential Aβ probes (for review, see Villemagne and Rowe[31]). Although selective tau imaging for in vivo NFT quantification is in the early stages of development, several Aβ radiotracers have found their way into human clinical trials.

Almost a decade after unsuccessful trials with anti-Aβ antibodies, Aβ imaging came to fruition with the first report of successful imaging in an AD patient with ^{18}F-FDDNP, a tracer claimed to bind both plaques and NFT.[32] Since then, human Aβ imaging studies have been conducted in AD patients, normal controls, and patients with other dementias using ^{11}C-labeled Pittsburgh compound B (^{11}C-PiB),[18] ^{18}F-florbetaben,[33] ^{18}F-flutemetamol,[34] ^{18}F-florbetapir,[35] and ^{18}F-AZD4694.[36]

^{11}C-labeled Pittsburgh Compound B

^{11}C-PiB, the most successful and widely used of the currently available Aβ tracers, has been shown to possess high affinity and high selectivity for fibrillar Aβ in plaques and in other Aβ-containing lesions.[37,38] Recent studies have shown that ^{11}C-PiB binds with high affinity to the N-terminally truncated and modified Aβ and AβN3-pyroglutamate species in senile plaques.[39] In vitro assessment of ^{3}H-PiB binding to white matter homogenates failed to show any specific binding.[40] ^{11}C-PiB is a derivative of thioflavin T, a fluorescent dye commonly used to assess fibrillization into β-sheet conformation; as such, ^{11}C-PiB has been shown to bind to a range of additional Aβ-containing lesions, including diffuse plaques and cerebral amyloid angiopathy (CAA),[41] as well as to Aβ oligomers—albeit with lower affinity.[42] ^{11}C-PiB also displayed lower affinity toward other misfolded proteins with a similar β-sheet secondary structure, such as α-synuclein[43] and tau.[41] Most importantly, these studies have shown that, at the concentrations achieved during a PET scan, ^{11}C-PiB cortical retention primarily reflects Aβ-related cerebral amyloidosis and not binding to Lewy bodies or NFT.[41,43,44] ^{11}C-PiB has consistently provided quantitative information on Aβ burden in vivo, contributing new insights into Aβ deposition in the brain, allowing earlier detection of AD pathology[18,19,37,45] and accurate differential diagnosis of the dementias.[19,46,47]

^{18}F-Labeled Radiotracers

The 20-minute radioactive decay half-life of carbon-11 (^{11}C) limits the use of ^{11}C-PiB to centers with an on-site cyclotron and ^{11}C radiochemistry expertise, making the cost of studies prohibitive for routine clinical use. To overcome these limitations, several Aβ tracers labeled with fluorine-18 (^{18}F) (half-life of 110 minutes) that permit centralized production and regional distribution have been developed and tested. Recent studies with the newly introduced ^{18}F-labeled Aβ-specific radiotracers, ^{18}F-florbetapir,[35,48] ^{18}F-florbetaben,[33,49,50] ^{18}F-flutemetamol,[51,52] and ^{18}F-AZD4694,[36] have been successfully replicating the results obtained with ^{11}C-PiB (**Fig. 1**).

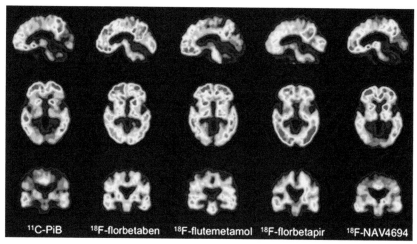

Fig. 1. Representative sagittal (*top row*), transaxial (*middle row*), and coronal (*bottom row*) PET images from AD patients obtained with different Aβ imaging radiotracers. From left to right, ^{11}C-PiB, ^{18}F-florbetaben, ^{18}F-flutemetamol, ^{18}F-florbetapir, and ^{18}F-NAV4694 (previously named AZD4694). The images show the typical pattern of tracer retention in AD, with the highest retention in frontal, temporal, posterior parietal and posterior cingulate cortices, reflecting Aβ plaque burden.

The dynamic range of ^{18}F-FDDNP cortical uptake is small, with only a 9% increase in mean cortical binding in AD compared with controls. Direct comparison of ^{18}F-FDDNP with ^{11}C-PiB showed limited dynamic range of ^{18}F-FDDNP[53] and in a longitudinal study was found less useful than ^{11}C-PiB and [18]F- FDG for examining disease progression.[54] ^{18}F-FDDNP remains the only Aβ tracer showing retention in the medial temporal cortex of AD patients and correlation with CSF tau.[53]

[18]F-florbetaben (also known as AV1 or BAY94-9172), synthesized by Kung and colleagues,[55] was the first ^{18}F-labeled specific brain amyloid tracer studied in humans with 50% to 70% higher cortical binding at 90 minutes' postinjection in AD subjects compared with age-matched controls and FTLD patients, with binding matching the reported postmortem distribution of Aβ plaques.[33] Recently completed phase II and phase III clinical studies further confirm these results,[49] and an ongoing longitudinal study in MCI subjects reports high predictive power for progression to AD.[56] ^{18}F-florbetaben binding is highly correlated with ^{11}C-PiB ($r = 0.97$, slope = 0.71),[57] and has been used to detect the presence or absence of AD pathology in the brain in subjects from a wide spectrum of neurodegenerative diseases.[50]

[18]F-florbetapir (also known as AV45) is another stilbene derivative also synthesized by Kung and colleagues[58] at the University of Pennsylvania. It has more rapid reversible binding characteristics, allowing scanning to commence 45 to 50 minutes after injection, similar to ^{11}C-PiB.[35] A phase III study in 59 patients established that ^{18}F-florbetapir has a sensitivity of 92% and a specificity of 100% for the detection of Aβ pathology.[59] ^{18}F-florbetapir studies in the same individuals have reported variable correlations with ^{11}C-PiB, with a linear correlation coefficient of $r = 0.77$ and a slope = 0.33[60] or a Spearman correlation ρ of 0.86 to 0.95 and slopes ranging from 0.59 to 0.64.[61] ^{18}F-florbetapir (as Amyvid) is the first radiotracer approved by the Food and Drug Administration for detection of Aβ in vivo.

[18]F-flutemetamol (also known as GE067)[62] has also completed phase III studies.[63] Phase I and phase II studies demonstrated that ^{18}F-flutemetamol can differentiate

between AD and healthy controls (HCs)[52] and that when combined with brain atrophy could be predictive of disease progression in MCI subjects.[64] ^{18}F-flutemetamol brain retention is also highly correlated with ^{11}C-PiB ($r = 0.91$, slope $= 0.90$).[52,64–66] Furthermore, there was a high correlation between Aβ burden as measured by ^{18}F-flutemetamol and by immunohistochemical assessment of brain biopsy tissue.[67,68]

Although the cortical retention of ^{18}F-florbetapir, ^{18}F-florbetaben, and ^{18}F-flutemetamol provides a clear separation of AD patients from HC subjects, the degree of cortical retention with ^{18}F-florbetapir and ^{18}F-florbetaben is lower than with ^{11}C-PiB,[57,60] showing a narrower dynamic range of standardized uptake value ratios that visually appears as a higher degree of nonspecific binding to white matter. Although the cortical retention of ^{18}F-flutemetamol is similar to that of ^{11}C-PiB, the nonspecific retention in white matter is much higher.[52] Although ^{11}C-PiB PET images in subjects with AD pathology usually clearly show high radiotracer retention in the gray matter in excess of that in subjacent white matter, these novel ^{18}F tracers frequently show loss of the normal gray–white matter demarcation as the predominant evidence of cortical Aβ deposition.[69]

^{18}F-AZD4694, recently renamed NAV4694, has yet to complete phase II trials but it has fast tracer kinetics, low nonspecific binding to white matter, and a wide dynamic range between HC and AD,[36] characteristics that are similar to ^{11}C-PiB. Initial clinical studies show a clear distinction in tracer retention between healthy elderly controls or FTLD patients and AD patients and high correlation with ^{11}C-PiB in a same subject comparison study ($r = 0.98$, slope $= 0.95$).[70]

AMYLOID IMAGING FINDINGS IN ALZHEIMER DISEASE

On visual inspection, amyloid scans in patients with AD show a typical regional brain distribution with highest binding in frontal, cingulate, precuneus, striatum, parietal, and lateral temporal cortices, whereas occipital, sensorimotor, and mesial temporal cortices are much less affected. Both quantitative and visual assessment of PET images present a pattern of radiotracer retention that seems to replicate the sequence of Aβ deposition found at autopsy,[71] with initial deposition in the orbitofrontal cortex, inferior temporal, cingulate gyrus, and precuneus followed by the remaining prefrontal cortex and lateral temporal and parietal cortices (**Fig. 2**). Multimodality studies in early AD have shown that the regional pattern of Aβ deposition is similar to the anatomy of the default network,[72] a specific, anatomically defined brain system responsible for internal modes of cognition, such as self-reflection processes, conscious resting state, or episodic memory retrieval,[73] an association that is present even in nondemented subjects.[74]

Carriers of mutations associated with familial AD,[75,76] differ in that high binding in the anterior striatum often precedes cortical binding. Patients with posterior cortical atrophy or CAA may show greater occipital binding than usually observed in sporadic AD but this is too variable to be of diagnostic value.

Longitudinal studies show not only that significant, albeit small, increases in Aβ deposition can be measured but also that these increases in Aβ deposition are present in the whole spectrum of cognitive stages, from cognitively unimpaired individuals to AD dementia patients.[77–80] Aβ accumulation has been observed on serial scans over several years in some individuals considered to have negative scans, with approximately 7% healthy elderly with a negative amyloid scan crossing the threshold for a positive scan in approximately 2.5 years.[81] Aβ accumulation is a slow process and the evidence suggests that it remains constant in the preclinical and prodromal stages of the disease in those individuals deemed to have high Aβ burdens while being

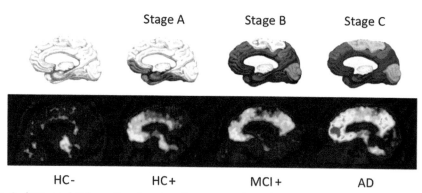

Stage A   Stage B   Stage C

HC−   HC+   MCI+   AD

Fig. 2. (*Top row*) Schematics showing the stages of Aβ deposition in the human brain as proposed by Braak and Braak. (*Bottom row*) Representative sagittal PET images showing the regional brain distribution of ^{11}C-PiB in 2 asymptomatic healthy age-matched controls, 1 with low (HC−) and 1 with high (HC+) Aβ burden, a subject classified as mild cognitive impairment (MCI+) with significant Aβ deposition in the brain, and an AD patient with even a higher Aβ burden in the brain. The pattern of PiB retention replicates the sequence of Aβ deposition described from postmortem studies. (*Data from* Braak H, Braak E. Frequency of stages of Alzheimer-related lesions in different age categories. Neurobiol Aging 1997;18:351–7.)

slightly higher at the early stages of AD.[80] In individuals with the highest Aβ burdens independent of clinical classification and also as AD progresses, the rates of Aβ deposition start to slow down, although not completely reaching a plateau.[79] This slower rate of Aβ deposition associated with disease progression might be attributed to a saturation of the process or, more likely, extensive neuronal death that precludes Aβ production.

POSTMORTEM CORRELATION WITH AMYLOID IMAGING

Although clinicopathologic studies have shown that the accuracy of clinical assessments for the diagnosis of AD ranges between 70% and 90%, depending on the specialization of the center, the regional retention of ^{11}C-PiB and the ^{18}F amyloid radiotracers is highly correlated with regional Aβ plaques as reported at autopsy or biopsy,[44,48,67,68,82–88] with a higher Aβ concentration in the frontal cortex than in hippocampus, consistent with previous reports on the distribution of amyloid plaques.[89,90] There have been some cases reported, however, of positive neuropathologic findings or a strong biomarker profile of AD and a negative PET scan. Three cases were in rare autosomal dominant gene mutation carriers.[91,92] In most cases of familial AD, there is prominent radiotracer binding to plaques. However, in 1 case of a novel APP mutation (E693Delta), where the mutant Aβ did not fibrillize in the same way as wild-type Aβ, and in 2 carriers of the Artic APP mutation, where atypical plaque morphology with ring-like plaques lacking a congophilic core were reported, amyloid scans were interpreted as negative. There have been 4 sporadic cases reported to date with plaques at autopsy but negative amyloid PET scans.[85,87,93,94] A nondemented patient with suspected normal pressure hydrocephalus had a frontal biopsy with plaques and a negative ^{11}C-PiB scan; another patient had cognitive decline with a CSF profile of AD but negative scan and 2.5 years later showed diffuse Aβ plaques with only minimal neuritic plaques and NFT pathology; a participant in the Baltimore Longitudinal Study of Aging[87] showed low global and regional ^{11}C-PiB retention despite moderate plaques at a neuropathologic examination that met

Consortium to Establish a Registry for Alzheimer's Disease [CERAD]) criteria for possible AD; and in 1 patient with both dementia with Lewy Bodies autopsy findings and focally frequent neocortical neuritic plaques that fulfilled CERAD criteria of definite AD but a ^{11}C-PiB scan 17 months earlier showed low binding. In this last case, the majority of plaques in postmortem tissue only labeled weakly with ^{11}C-PiB and ^{3}H-PiB, suggesting low fibrillar Aβ content.

These cases illustrate the possibility that different conformations of Aβ deposits may affect the binding of tracers and that Aβ imaging may not recognize all types of Aβ pathologies with equal sensitivity.

Reassuringly, with completion of the phase III trials for florbetapir, florbetaben, and flutemetamol, data on 207 imaged patients, who have been characterized by histopathologic examination on postmortem or brain biopsy specimens, have been presented that confirm that amyloid imaging with PET accurately reflects the concentration of dense plaques. Sensitivity for detection of amyloid plaque sufficient to meet CERAD criteria for probable AD ranged from 86% to 100%, with specificity ranging from 92% to 100%. These results confirm the ability of amyloid imaging to detect plaques and that patients with a negative amyloid scan are unlikely to have AD.

AMYLOID IMAGING IN AGING AND MILD COGNITIVE IMPAIRMENT

Approximately 25% to 35% of elderly subjects performing within normal age and education corrected limits on cognitive tests have high cortical ^{11}C-PiB retention, predominantly in the prefrontal and posterior cingulate/precuneus regions.[45,95–98] These findings are in agreement with postmortem reports that approximately 25% of nondemented older individuals over the age of 75 have Aβ plaques.[99,100] Aβ deposition in these nondemented individuals might reflect the preclinical stage of AD. Furthermore, the prevalence of subjects with high ^{11}C-PiB retention increases each decade at the same rate as the reported prevalence of plaques in nondemented subjects in autopsy studies.[98] Although cross-sectional examination of these controls essentially show no significant differences in cognition, significant cognitive differences in women were reported.[101] More recently, Sperling and colleagues[102] reported that high Aβ deposition in the brain was correlated with lower immediate and delayed memory scores in otherwise healthy controls. The detection of Aβ pathology at the presymptomatic stage is of crucial importance, because if this group truly represents the preclinical stage of AD, it is precisely the group that may benefit the most from therapies aimed at reducing or eliminating Aβ from the brain before irreversible neuronal or synaptic loss occurs.

Individuals fulfilling criteria for MCI are a heterogeneous group with a wide spectrum of underlying pathologies.[20,103] Approximately 40% to 60% of carefully characterized subjects with MCI subsequently progress to meet criteria for AD over a 3-year to 4-year period.[20,21,104] Aβ imaging has proved useful in identifying MCI individuals with and without AD pathology. Approximately 50% to 70% of the subjects classified as MCI have high cortical ^{11}C-PiB retention.[38,96,105–108] Most subjects classified as nonamnestic MCI show low Aβ levels in the brain.[107,108]

To date, the relationship between Aβ deposition and the development of clinical symptoms is not fully understood. Although Aβ burden as assessed by PET does not correlate with measures of memory impairment in established clinical AD, it does correlate with memory impairment in nondemented subjects (ie, MCI combined with healthy older individuals).[108] In subjects with MCI, this Aβ-related impairment is believed mediated through hippocampal atrophy,[96] while modulated by cognitive reserve[109,110] and glucose metabolism,[111] although at the AD stage there is no longer correlation between glucose metabolism, cognition, and Aβ burden.[112]

Longitudinal studies are helping in clarify the relationship between Aβ burden and cognitive decline in healthy individuals and MCI subjects. High ^{11}C-PiB cortical retention in nondemented elderly subjects is associated with a greater risk of cognitive decline. For example, the evaluation of either the cognitive trajectories[113,114] or changes in cognition prospectively[80,115,116] shows that individuals with substantial Aβ deposition are more likely to present with cognitive decline. Aggregating the results from recently reported longitudinal studies reveals that 65% of MCI subjects with marked ^{11}C-PiB retention progressed to AD over 2 to 3 years, showing that MCI subjects with high Aβ deposition in the brain are more than 10 times more likely to progress to AD than those with low Aβ deposition, highlighting the clinical relevance and potential impact on patient management of Aβ imaging.[80,105,117–119] The observations that ^{11}C-PiB retention in nondemented individuals relates to episodic memory impairment, one of the earliest clinical symptoms of AD, and that extensive Aβ deposition is associated with a significantly higher risk of cognitive decline in HC and with progression from MCI to AD, emphasizes the nonbenign nature of Aβ deposition and supports the hypothesis that Aβ deposition occurs well before the onset of symptoms, further suggesting that early disease-specific therapeutic intervention at the presymptomatic stage might be the most promising approach to either delay onset or halt disease progression.[120]

The lack of a strong association between Aβ deposition and measures of cognition, synaptic activity, and neurodegeneration in AD, in addition to the evidence of Aβ deposition in a high percentage of MCI and asymptomatic HC, suggests that Aβ is an early and necessary, although not sufficient, cause for cognitive decline in AD, indicating the involvement of other downstream mechanisms, likely triggered by Aβ, such as NFT formation, synaptic failure, and eventually neuronal loss. Age, years of education, occupational level, and brain volume, under the umbrella of cognitive reserve, seem to have a modulatory role between cognition and Aβ deposition.[110,121,122]

COMPARISON OF AMYLOID IMAGING TO OTHER INVESTIGATIONS

Fluorodeoxyglucose PET Imaging of Cerebral Glucose Metabolism

Visual assessment of PET images by clinicians blinded to clinical status has demonstrated that ^{11}C-PiB was more accurate than ^{18}F-FDG in distinguishing AD from HC[123] and slightly better than ^{18}F-FDG in differentiating AD from FTLD.[124] Similarly, Aβ imaging outperforms ^{18}F-FDG at identifying MCI subtypes.[107]

Although some reports found no association between ^{18}F-FDG and ^{11}C-PiB in AD,[112] others found an inverse correlation between them in temporal and parietal cortices,[111] but no correlation has been shown in the frontal lobe. A possible explanation for this dissociation is that there are compensatory mechanisms, such as upregulation of choline acetyltransferase in the frontal lobe of MCI individuals and mild AD patients[125,126] that might delay the manifestation of synaptic dysfunction; therefore, no frontal hypometabolism is observed on ^{18}F-FDG. Glucose metabolism in the frontal lobe eventually decreases as the disease progresses, and the characteristic temporoparietal pattern of AD becomes less apparent.[127] Converse to what is observed in the frontal area, in AD patients, choline acetyltransferase is significantly decreased in the posterior cingulate gyrus,[128] a region of marked and early Aβ deposition and substantial hypometabolism.[74]

Cerebrospinal Fluid Analysis

Analysis of CSF allows simultaneous measurement of the concentration of the 2 main hallmarks of AD, Aβ and tau. It has been reported to be highly accurate in the diagnosis of AD as well as in predicting cognitive decline.[129–132] The typical CSF profile in AD is low $A\beta_{1-42}$ and high total tau and phosphorylated tau. Although there is no correlation between ^{11}C-PiB retention and CSF total tau or phosphorylated tau,[133,134] several studies have reported a strong inverse correlation between $A\beta$ deposition in the brain as measured by ^{11}C-PiB and CSF $A\beta_{1-42}$.[105,135–138] Both high ^{11}C-PiB retention and low CSF $A\beta_{1-42}$ have been observed in cognitively unimpaired individuals, probably reflecting $A\beta$ deposition years before the manifestation of the AD phenotype. Large population studies, such as the *Alzheimer's Disease Neuroimaging Initiative*,[139,140] will further validate the value of $A\beta$ imaging and CSF assessments as antecedent biomarkers of AD.

MRI

Although $A\beta$ imaging or CSF $A\beta$ provides information on $A\beta$ pathology, CSF tau quantification, ^{18}F-FDG, and structural MRI provide information related to the neurodegenerative process.[14] Hippocampal and cortical gray matter atrophy along with ventricular enlargement are typical MRI findings in AD and MCI.[141] $A\beta$ deposition is associated with regional cerebral atrophy as measured by MRI[142–145] and correlates with the rates of cerebral atrophy.[143,146] The data suggest that the relationship between $A\beta$ deposition and cortical atrophy is sequential, where $A\beta$ deposition precedes synaptic dysfunction and neuronal loss,[74,145,147] with the latter subsequently apparent as progressive atrophy on structural imaging.[143] Normal elderly persons with high $A\beta$ deposition show a significantly higher rate of atrophy in the temporal and posterior cingulate cortices compared with those with low $A\beta$ burden.[148]

GENETIC RISK AND OTHER PREDISPOSING FACTORS FOR BRAIN AMYLOID

Age is the strongest risk factor in sporadic AD, with the prevalence of the disease increasing exponentially with age. These risks are increased in the presence of the ApoE ε4 allele.[149] Both risk factors have been directly associated with $A\beta$ burden as measured by PET.[97,98]

Examination of ApoE ε4 allele status revealed that, independent of clinical classification, ε4 carriers have significantly higher ^{11}C-PiB retention than non–ε4 carriers, further emphasizing the crucial role that ApoE plays in the metabolism of $A\beta$. In patients who have established dementia due to AD, however, there is no significant difference in $A\beta$ burden between ε4 carriers and non–ε4 carriers[18,19,150,151] nor does there seem to be faster rate of amyloid accumulation in nondemented carriers, suggesting that ε4 confers earlier onset of accumulation.

Both symptomatic and asymptomatic individual carriers of mutations within the APP or presenilin 1 or presenilin 2 gene associated with familial AD have high and early ^{11}C-PiB retention in the caudate nuclei, retention that seems independent of mutation type or disease severity.[75,76] Larger multicenter studies are helping elucidate the value of several biomarkers in these autosomal mutation carriers, assessment that might lead to better targeted, disease-specific therapeutic strategies.[152]

Although a similar pattern of $A\beta$ deposition as seen in AD has been reported in older adults with Down syndrome,[153] a completely different pattern of ^{11}C-PiB retention was observed in a mutation carrier of familial British dementia.[154]

DIFFERENTIAL DIAGNOSIS OF DEMENTIA WITH AMYLOID IMAGING

Although lower than in AD, similar patterns of ^{11}C-PiB retention are usually observed in DLB.[19,155,156] Cortical ^{11}C-PiB retention is also elevated in subjects diagnosed with cerebral amyloid angiopathy (CAA),[157] although there is usually no cortical ^{11}C-PiB retention in patients with FTLD.[19,47,158,159]

The contribution of Aβ to the development of Lewy body diseases remains unclear, but cortical Aβ deposits are associated with extensive α-synuclein lesions and higher levels of insoluble α-synuclein protein[160] as well as exacerbation of neuronal injury.[161] Although Aβ imaging cannot contribute to the differential diagnosis between AD and DLB, it may have prognostic relevance in these Lewy body diseases. For example, similar to what has been reported for Parkinson's disease dementia (PDD), where higher Aβ burden was associated with a shorter prodromal phase before dementia,[162] Aβ burden in DLB patients was inversely correlated with the interval from onset of cognitive impairment to the full development of the DLB phenotype.[19]

FTLD is a syndrome that can also be clinically difficult to distinguish from early-onset AD, especially at the initial stages of the disease. Aβ deposition is not a pathologic trait of FTLD. Based on clinical phenotype, FTLD has been categorized mainly into 2 classes: behavioral variant of FTLD, with distinct changes in behavior and personality with little effect on language functions, and progressive aphasias (comprised by semantic dementia and progressive nonfluent aphasia).[163] Approximately one-third of progressive aphasia, however, is due to a variant of AD. These cases have distinct clinical features and have been termed, *logopenic aphasia*, and have positive amyloid scans that are largely indistinguishable from sporadic AD despite the focal nature of the cognitive deficit.[164]

Aβ imaging has been helpful in the differential diagnosis between FTLD and AD.[19,47,158,159] Furthermore, Aβ imaging has been used to ascertain the absence of AD pathology in the different FTLD aphasias.[158,164,165] Despite displaying similar specificities, the diagnostic performance of Aβ imaging proved more sensitive for the diagnosis of FTLD than ^{18}F-FDG.[124]

No cortical ^{11}C-PiB retention was observed in 2 sporadic Creutzfeldt-Jakob disease cases.[88]

APPROPRIATE USE OF AMYLOID IMAGING

[18]F-florbetapir was recently approved by the Food and Drug Administration for the detection of amyloid in the brain and is now available for clinical use in the United States. Several other amyloid imaging tracers are likely to also become available over the next few years. Appropriate clinical use criteria are needed for 2 reasons: (1) there is the potential to do harm if the scans are performed in inappropriate circumstances or are poorly read or if the significance of the results is not correctly applied to the clinical context and (2) these investigations are expensive and the cost-benefit ratio to society must be considered. An example of the potential to do harm is to perform an amyloid scan in an individual who is cognitively intact and, if the result is positive, to inform that person that he/she has AD. Positive scans are found in 30% of cognitively normal persons over the age of 70 years and there is insufficient follow-up data available to date to assess the potential risk and likely time of onset of cognitive decline and dementia in an individual with a positive scan. It is known that the rate of amyloid accumulation is slow and it takes 15 to 20 years for amyloid plaque density to increase from when first detectable by amyloid scan to the level typically found in patients with dementia due to AD. Consequently, the majority of normal elderly people with a positive scan are still normal in 5 and perhaps 10 years time. Many die from other illnesses having never developed dementia. Premature or inappropriate labeling of an individual with the diagnosis of AD is likely to have detrimental psychological, social, employment, financial, and lifestyle consequences. Harm could also be done to a patient with coexistent cognitive complaints and depression by denying appropriate therapy. If a scan is performed and found positive, the risk of

incidental amyloid must be taken into consideration when planning management because it may be inappropriate and harmful to not provide treatment of depression. Other markers to support a diagnosis of AD are needed in this instance, such as the typical episodic memory dominant AD pattern of cognitive impairment, hippocampal atrophy on MRI, or parietotemporal hypometabolism on FDG-PET. In this situation, the greater value of an amyloid scan may be from a negative result to exclude AD and encourage a more vigorous evaluation of alternative diagnoses and treatment of depression. These examples illustrate that the result of an amyloid scan in isolation can be misleading and the scan should be just one component of a comprehensive evaluation performed by a physician with expertise in the evaluation of cognitive complaints and dementia.

The lack of an effective therapy or intervention proved to prevent, delay, or slow the progression of AD further complicates the appropriate use of amyloid imaging, particularly when looking at cost effectiveness. Clinicians must weigh the benefits before ordering a test that costs several thousand dollars when it is unlikely to improve the

---

Box 1
Appropriate use criteria as defined by the Society of Nuclear Medicine and Molecular Imaging and the Alzheimer's Association joint Amyloid Imaging Task Force 2012

Amyloid imaging is appropriate in the situations listed below as 1 to 3 for individuals with all of the following characteristics:

a. a cognitive complaint with objectively confirmed impairment;

b. Alzheimer's disease as a possible diagnosis, but when the diagnosis is uncertain after a comprehensive evaluation by a dementia expert;

c. when knowledge of the presence or absence of amyloid-beta pathology is expected to increase diagnostic certainty and alter management.

Appropriate situations:

1. Patients with persistent or progressive unexplained mild cognitive impairment

2. Patients satisfying core clinical criteria for possible Alzheimer's disease but not probable AD because of unclear clinical presentation, either atypical clinical course or etiologically mixed presentation

3. Patients with progressive dementia and atypically early age of onset (defined as 65 years or less in age)

Amyloid imaging is inappropriate in the situations listed:

1. Patients with core clinical criteria for probable Alzheimer's disease with typical age of onset

2. To determine dementia severity

3. Solely based on a positive family history of dementia or presence of ApoE4

4. Patients with a cognitive complaint that is unconfirmed on clinical examination

5. In lieu of genotyping for suspected autosomal mutation carriers

6. In asymptomatic individuals

7. Non-medical usage (e.g. legal, insurance coverage, or employment screening)

From Johnson KA, Minoshima S, Bohnen NI, et al. Appropriate use criteria for amyloid PET: a report of the Amyloid Imaging Task Force, the Society of Nuclear Medicine and Molecular Imaging, and the Alzheimer's Association. Alzheimers Dement 2013;9:e.1–16; with permission.

long-term outcome for a patient. Unless there is a reasonable likelihood of improved diagnostic accuracy and management change for a particular patient, the test should not be ordered.

A joint task force of the Society of Nuclear Medicine and Molecular Imaging and the Alzheimer's Association undertook a review, in late 2012, of the available literature and sought expert opinion to define appropriate use criteria for amyloid imaging. The conclusions of this task force are listed in **Box 1**. At the time of this assessment, however, there were few data available on appropriate clinical use or comparative effectiveness of amyloid imaging, so these recommendations may change as data emerge and need to be completely redefined should an effective therapy for prevention or treatment for AD emerge.

As new therapies enter clinical trials, the role of Aβ imaging in vivo is becoming increasingly crucial. Aβ imaging allows the in vivo assessment of brain Aβ pathology and its changes over time, providing highly accurate, reliable, and reproducible quantitative statements of regional or global Aβ burden in the brain. As discussed previously, therapies, especially those targeting irreversible neurodegenerative processes, have a better chance to succeed if applied early, making early detection of the underlying pathologic process important. Therefore, Aβ imaging is an ideal tool for the selection of adequate candidates for anti-Aβ therapeutic trials while also monitoring—and potentially predicting—treatment response, thus aiding in reducing sample size, minimizing cost while maximizing outcomes. Longitudinal studies support the growing consensus that for anti-Aβ therapy to be effective, it may need to be given early in the course of the disease, perhaps even before symptoms appear,[120] and that downstream mechanisms may also need to be addressed to successfully prevent the development of AD. Furthermore, the slow rate of Aβ deposition indicates that the time window for altering Aβ accumulation before the full manifestation of the clinical phenotype may be wide.[80]

ACKNOWLEDGMENTS

We thank Professor Michael Woodward, Dr John Merory, Dr Peter Drysdale, Dr Gordon Chan, Dr Kenneth Young, Dr Sylvia Gong, Dr Greg Savage, Dr Paul Maruff, Dr David Darby, Ms Fiona Lamb, Mr Sean Thronton, Ms Mary Kate Danaher, Ms Joanne Robertson, and the Brain Research Institute for their assistance with this study.

REFERENCES

1. Masters CL, Cappai R, Barnham KJ, et al. Molecular mechanisms for Alzheimer's disease: implications for neuroimaging and therapeutics. J Neurochem 2006;97: 1700–25.
2. Khachaturian ZS. Diagnosis of Alzheimer's disease. Arch Neurol 1985;42: 1097–105.
3. Jellinger K. Morphology of Alzheimer disease and related disorders. In: Maurer K, et al, editors. Alzheimer disease: epidemiology, neuropathology, neurochemistry, and clinics. Berlin: Springer-Verlag; 1990. p. 61–77.
4. Masters CL, Beyreuther K. The neuropathology of Alzheimer's disease in the year 2005. In: Beal MF, et al, editors. Neurodegenerative diseases: neurobiology, pathogenesis and therapeutics. Cambridge (England): Cambridge University Press; 2005. p. 433–40.
5. Jellinger KA, Bancher C. Neuropathology of Alzheimer's disease: a critical update. J Neural Transm Suppl 1998;54:77–95.

6. Masters CL, Simms G, Weinman NA, et al. Amyloid plaque core protein in Alzheimer disease and Down syndrome. Proc Natl Acad Sci U S A 1985;82:4245–9.
7. Cappai R, White AR. Amyloid beta. Int J Biochem Cell Biol 1999;31:885–9.
8. Villemagne VL, Cappai R, Barnham KJ, et al. The Aβ centric pathway of Alzheimer's disease. In: Barrow CJ, Small BJ, editors. Abeta peptide and Alzheimer's Disease. London: Springer-Verlag; 2006. p. 5–32.
9. Hardy J. Amyloid, the presenilins and Alzheimer's disease. Trends Neurosci 1997;20:154–9.
10. McKhann G, Drachman D, Folstein M, et al. Clinical diagnosis of Alzheimer's Disease: report of the NINCDS-ADRDA Work Group under the auspices of Department of Health and Human Services Task Force on Alzheimer's disease. Neurology 1984;34:939–44.
11. Knopman DS, DeKosky ST, Cummings JL, et al. Practice parameter: Diagnosis of dementia (an evidence based review). Report of the Quality Standards Subcommittee of the American Academy of Neurology. Neurology 2001;56: 1143–53.
12. McKhann GM, Knopman DS, Chertkow H, et al. The diagnosis of dementia due to Alzheimer's disease: recommendations from the National Institute on Aging-Alzheimer's Association workgroups on diagnostic guidelines for Alzheimer's disease. Alzheimers Dement 2011;7:263–9.
13. Clark CM, Davatzikos C, Borthakur A, et al. Biomarkers for early detection of Alzheimer pathology. Neurosignals 2008;16:11–8.
14. Jack CR Jr, Knopman DS, Jagust WJ, et al. Hypothetical model of dynamic biomarkers of the Alzheimer's pathological cascade. Lancet Neurol 2010;9: 119–28.
15. de Leon MJ, Convit A, DeSanti S, et al. Contribution of structural neuroimaging to the early diagnosis of Alzheimer's disease. Int Psychogeriatr 1997;9:183–90 [discussion: 247–52].
16. Xu Y, Jack CR Jr, O'Brien PC, et al. Usefulness of MRI measures of entorhinal cortex versus hippocampus in AD. Neurology 2000;54:1760–7.
17. Silverman DH, Small GW, Chang CY, et al. Positron emission tomography in evaluation of dementia: regional brain metabolism and long-term outcome. JAMA 2001;286:2120–7.
18. Klunk WE, Engler H, Nordberg A, et al. Imaging brain amyloid in Alzheimer's disease with Pittsburgh Compound-B. Ann Neurol 2004;55:306–19.
19. Rowe CC, Ng S, Ackermann U, et al. Imaging beta-amyloid burden in aging and dementia. Neurology 2007;68:1718–25.
20. Petersen RC. Mild cognitive impairment: transition between aging and Alzheimer's disease. Neurologia 2000;15:93–101.
21. Petersen RC, Smith GE, Waring SC, et al. Mild cognitive impairment: clinical characterization and outcome. Arch Neurol 1999;56:303–8.
22. Dubois B, Feldman HH, Jacova C, et al. Revising the definition of Alzheimer's disease: a new lexicon. Lancet Neurol 2010;9:1118–27.
23. Albert MS, Dekosky ST, Dickson D, et al. The diagnosis of mild cognitive impairment due to Alzheimer's disease: recommendations from the National Institute on Aging-Alzheimer's Association workgroups on diagnostic guidelines for Alzheimer's disease. Alzheimers Dement 2011;7:270–9.
24. Petersen RC. Mild cognitive impairment: current research and clinical implications. Semin Neurol 2007;27:22–31.
25. Phelps ME. PET: the merging of biology and imaging into molecular imaging. J Nucl Med 2000;41:661–81.

26. Mathis CA, Klunk WE, Price JC, et al. Imaging technology for neurodegenerative diseases: progress toward detection of specific pathologies. Arch Neurol 2005; 62:196–200.

27. Villemagne VL, Rowe CC, Macfarlane S, et al. Imaginem oblivionis: the prospects of neuroimaging for early detection of Alzheimer's disease. J Clin Neurosci 2005;12:221–30.

28. Laruelle M, Slifstein M, Huang Y. Relationships between radiotracer properties and image quality in molecular imaging of the brain with positron emission tomography. Mol Imaging Biol 2003;5:363–75.

29. Nordberg A. PET imaging of amyloid in Alzheimer's disease. Lancet Neurol 2004;3:519–27.

30. Pike VW. PET radiotracers: crossing the blood-brain barrier and surviving metabolism. Trends Pharmacol Sci 2009;30:431–40.

31. Villemagne VL, Rowe CC. Amyloid ligands for dementia. PET Clin 2010;5:33–53.

32. Shoghi-Jadid K, Small GW, Agdeppa ED, et al. Localization of neurofibrillary tangles and beta-amyloid plaques in the brains of living patients with Alzheimer disease. Am J Geriatr Psychiatry 2002;10:24–35.

33. Rowe CC, Ackerman U, Browne W, et al. Imaging of amyloid beta in Alzheimer's disease with (18)F-BAY94-9172, a novel PET tracer: proof of mechanism. Lancet Neurol 2008;7:129–35.

34. Serdons K, Terwinghe C, Vermaelen P, et al. Synthesis and evaluation of (18)F-labeled 2-phenylbenzothiazoles as positron emission tomography imaging agents for amyloid plaques in Alzheimer's disease. J Med Chem 2009;52: 1428–37.

35. Wong DF, Rosenberg PB, Zhou Y, et al. In vivo imaging of amyloid deposition in Alzheimer disease using the radioligand 18F-AV-45 (florbetapir [corrected] F 18). J Nucl Med 2010;51:913–20.

36. Cselenyi Z, Jonhagen ME, Forsberg A, et al. Clinical Validation of 18F-AZD4694, an Amyloid-beta-Specific PET Radioligand. J Nucl Med 2012;53:415–24.

37. Cohen AD, Rabinovici GD, Mathis CA, et al. Using Pittsburgh compound B for in vivo PET imaging of fibrillar amyloid-beta. Adv Pharmacol 2012;64:27–81.

38. Price JC, Klunk WE, Lopresti BJ, et al. Kinetic modeling of amyloid binding in humans using PET imaging and Pittsburgh Compound-B. J Cereb Blood Flow Metab 2005;25:1528–47.

39. Maeda J, Ji B, Irie T, et al. Longitudinal, quantitative assessment of amyloid, neuroinflammation, and anti-amyloid treatment in a living mouse model of Alzheimer's disease enabled by positron emission tomography. J Neurosci 2007; 27:10957–68.

40. Fodero-Tavoletti MT, Rowe CC, McLean CA, et al. Characterization of PiB binding to white matter in Alzheimer disease and other dementias. J Nucl Med 2009;50:198–204.

41. Lockhart A, Lamb JR, Osredkar T, et al. PIB is a non-specific imaging marker of amyloid-beta (Abeta) peptide-related cerebral amyloidosis. Brain 2007;130: 2607–15.

42. Maezawa I, Hong HS, Liu R, et al. Congo red and thioflavin-T analogs detect Abeta oligomers. J Neurochem 2008;104:457–68.

43. Fodero-Tavoletti MT, Smith DP, McLean CA, et al. In vitro characterization of Pittsburgh compound-B binding to Lewy bodies. J Neurosci 2007;27:10365–71.

44. Ikonomovic MD, Klunk WE, Abrahamson EE, et al. Post-mortem correlates of in vivo PiB-PET amyloid imaging in a typical case of Alzheimer's disease. Brain 2008;131:1630–45.

45. Mintun MA, Larossa GN, Sheline YI, et al. [11C]PIB in a nondemented population: potential antecedent marker of Alzheimer disease. Neurology 2006;67: 446–52.

46. Ng SY, Villemagne VL, Masters CL, et al. Evaluating atypical dementia syndromes using positron emission tomography with carbon 11 labeled Pittsburgh Compound B. Arch Neurol 2007;64:1140–4.

47. Rabinovici GD, Furst AJ, O'Neil JP, et al. 11C-PIB PET imaging in Alzheimer disease and frontotemporal lobar degeneration. Neurology 2007;68:1205–12.

48. Clark CM, Schneider JA, Bedell BJ, et al. Use of florbetapir-PET for imaging beta-amyloid pathology. JAMA 2011;305:275–83.

49. Barthel H, Gertz HJ, Dresel S, et al. Cerebral amyloid-beta PET with florbetaben ((18)F) in patients with Alzheimer's disease and healthy controls: a multicentre phase 2 diagnostic study. Lancet Neurol 2011;10:424–35.

50. Villemagne VL, Ong K, Mulligan RS, et al. Amyloid Imaging with 18F-Florbetaben in Alzheimer disease and other dementias. J Nucl Med 2011;52:1210–7.

51. Nelissen N, Van Laere K, Thurfjell L, et al. Phase 1 study of the Pittsburgh compound B derivative 18F-flutemetamol in healthy volunteers and patients with probable Alzheimer disease. J Nucl Med 2009;50:1251–9.

52. Vandenberghe R, Van Laere K, Ivanoiu A, et al. 18F-flutemetamol amyloid imaging in Alzheimer disease and mild cognitive impairment: a phase 2 trial. Ann Neurol 2010;68:319–29.

53. Tolboom N, Yaqub M, van der Flier WM, et al. Detection of Alzheimer pathology in vivo using both 11C-PIB and 18F-FDDNP PET. J Nucl Med 2009;50:191–7.

54. Ossenkoppele R, Tolboom N, Foster-Dingley JC, et al. Longitudinal imaging of Alzheimer pathology using [11C]PIB, [18F]FDDNP and [18F]FDG PET. Eur J Nucl Med Mol Imaging 2012;39:990–1000.

55. Zhang W, Oya S, Kung MP, et al. F-18 stilbenes as PET imaging agents for detecting beta-amyloid plaques in the brain. J Med Chem 2005;48:5980–8.

56. Ong K, Villemagne VL, Lamngon N, et al. Assessment of Aβ Deposition in Mild Cognitive Impairment with 18F-Florbetaben. Alzheimers Dement 2010;6:S26.

57. Villemagne VL, Mulligan RS, Pejoska S, et al. Comparison of (11)C-PiB and (18) F-florbetaben for Aβ imaging in ageing and Alzheimer's disease. Eur J Nucl Med Mol Imaging 2012;39:983–9.

58. Zhang W, Oya S, Kung MP, et al. F-18 Polyethyleneglycol stilbenes as PET imaging agents targeting Abeta aggregates in the brain. Nucl Med Biol 2005; 32:799–809.

59. Clark CM, Pontecorvo MJ, Beach TG, et al. Cerebral PET with florbetapir compared with neuropathology at autopsy for detection of neuritic amyloid-beta plaques: a prospective cohort study. Lancet Neurol 2012;11:669–78.

60. Wolk DA, Zhang Z, Boudhar S, et al. Amyloid imaging in Alzheimer's disease: comparison of florbetapir and Pittsburgh compound-B positron emission tomography. J Neurol Neurosurg Psychiatry 2012;83:923–6.

61. Landau SM, Breault C, Joshi AD, et al. Amyloid-beta imaging with Pittsburgh compound B and florbetapir: comparing radiotracers and quantification methods. J Nucl Med 2012. http://dx.doi.org/10.2967/jnumed.112.109009.

62. Serdons K, Verduyckt T, Vanderghinste D, et al. Synthesis of 18F-labelled 2-(4'-fluorophenyl)-1,3-benzothiazole and evaluation as amyloid imaging agent in comparison with [11C]PIB. Bioorg Med Chem Lett 2009;19:602–5.

63. Buckley C, Ikonomovic M, Smith A, et al. Flutemetamol F 18 injection PET images reflect brain beta-amyloid levels. Alzheimers Dement 2012;8:P90.

64. Thurfjell L, Lotjonen J, Lundqvist R, et al. Combination of biomarkers: PET [18F] flutemetamol imaging and structural MRI in dementia and mild cognitive impairment. Neurodegener Dis 2012;10:246–9.

65. Duara R, Loewenstein DA, Shen Q, et al. Amyloid positron emission tomography with (18)F-flutemetamol and structural magnetic resonance imaging in the classification of mild cognitive impairment and Alzheimer's disease. Alzheimers Dement 2012. [Epub ahead of print].

66. Vandenberghe R, Nelissen N, Salmon E, et al. Binary classification of (18)F-flutemetamol PET using machine learning: comparison with visual reads and structural MRI. Neuroimage 2013;64:517–25.

67. Wolk DA, Grachev ID, Buckley C, et al. Association between in vivo fluorine 18-labeled flutemetamol amyloid positron emission tomography imaging and in vivo cerebral cortical histopathology. Arch Neurol 2011;68:1398–403.

68. Wong DF, Moghekar AR, Rigamonti D, et al. An in vivo evaluation of cerebral cortical amyloid with [(18)F]flutemetamol using positron emission tomography compared with parietal biopsy samples in living normal pressure hydrocephalus patients. Mol Imaging Biol 2012. [Epub ahead of print].

69. Rowe CC, Villemagne VL. Brain amyloid imaging. J Nucl Med 2011;52:1733–40.

70. Rowe CC, Pejoska S, Mulligan RS, et al. Head to head comparison of 11C-PiB and 18F-AZD4694 (NAV4694) for β-amyloid imaging in ageing and dementia. J Nucl Med 2013. [in press].

71. Braak H, Braak E. Frequency of stages of Alzheimer-related lesions in different age categories. Neurobiol Aging 1997;18:351–7.

72. Buckner RL, Snyder AZ, Shannon BJ, et al. Molecular, structural, and functional characterization of Alzheimer's disease: evidence for a relationship between default activity, amyloid, and memory. J Neurosci 2005;25:7709–17.

73. Buckner RL, Andrews-Hanna JR, Schacter DL. The brain's default network: anatomy, function, and relevance to disease. Ann N Y Acad Sci 2008;1124: 1–38.

74. Drzezga A, Becker JA, Van Dijk KR, et al. Neuronal dysfunction and disconnection of cortical hubs in non-demented subjects with elevated amyloid burden. Brain 2011;134:1635–46.

75. Klunk WE, Price JC, Mathis CA, et al. Amyloid deposition begins in the striatum of presenilin-1 mutation carriers from two unrelated pedigrees. J Neurosci 2007; 27:6174–84.

76. Villemagne VL, Ataka S, Mizuno T, et al. High striatal amyloid beta-peptide deposition across different autosomal Alzheimer disease mutation types. Arch Neurol 2009;66:1537–44.

77. Engler H, Forsberg A, Almkvist O, et al. Two-year follow-up of amyloid deposition in patients with Alzheimer's disease. Brain 2006;129:2856–66.

78. Jack CR Jr, Lowe VJ, Weigand SD, et al. Serial PIB and MRI in normal, mild cognitive impairment and Alzheimer's disease: implications for sequence of pathological events in Alzheimer's disease. Brain 2009;132:1355–65.

79. Villain N, Chetelat G, Grassiot B, et al. Regional dynamics of amyloid-beta deposition in healthy elderly, mild cognitive impairment and Alzheimer's disease: a voxelwise PiB-PET longitudinal study. Brain 2012;135:2126–39.

80. Villemagne VL, Pike KE, Chetelat G, et al. Longitudinal assessment of Aβ and cognition in aging and Alzheimer disease. Ann Neurol 2011;69:181–92.

81. Vlassenko AG, Mintun MA, Xiong C, et al. Amyloid-beta plaque growth in cognitively normal adults: longitudinal [11C]Pittsburgh compound B data. Ann Neurol 2011;70:857–61.

82. Bacskai BJ, Frosch MP, Freeman SH, et al. Molecular imaging with Pittsburgh Compound B confirmed at autopsy: a case report. Arch Neurol 2007;64: 431–4.
83. Burack MA, Hartlein J, Flores HP, et al. In vivo amyloid imaging in autopsy-confirmed Parkinson disease with dementia. Neurology 2010;74:77–84.
84. Kadir A, Marutle A, Gonzalez D, et al. Positron emission tomography imaging and clinical progression in relation to molecular pathology in the first Pittsburgh Compound B positron emission tomography patient with Alzheimer's disease. Brain 2011;134:301–17.
85. Leinonen V, Alafuzoff I, Aalto S, et al. Assessment of beta-amyloid in a frontal cortical brain biopsy specimen and by positron emission tomography with carbon 11-labeled Pittsburgh Compound B. Arch Neurol 2008;65:1304–9.
86. Sabbagh MN, Fleisher A, Chen K, et al. Positron emission tomography and neuropathologic estimates of fibrillar amyloid-beta in a patient with Down syndrome and Alzheimer disease. Arch Neurol 2011;68:1461–6.
87. Sojkova J, Driscoll I, Iacono D, et al. In vivo fibrillar beta-amyloid detected using [11C]PiB positron emission tomography and neuropathologic assessment in older adults. Arch Neurol 2011;68:232–40.
88. Villemagne VL, McLean CA, Reardon K, et al. 11C-PiB PET studies in typical sporadic Creutzfeldt-Jakob disease. J Neurol Neurosurg Psychiatry 2009;80: 998–1001.
89. Arnold SE, Han LY, Clark CM, et al. Quantitative neurohistological features of frontotemporal degeneration. Neurobiol Aging 2000;21:913–9.
90. Naslund J, Haroutunian V, Mohs R, et al. Correlation between elevated levels of amyloid beta-peptide in the brain and cognitive decline. JAMA 2000;283: 1571–7.
91. Schöll M, Almqvist O, Graff C, et al. Amyloid imaging in members of a family harbouring the Arctic mutation. Alzheimers Dement 2011;7(Suppl 1):303.
92. Tomiyama T, Nagata T, Shimada H, et al. A new amyloid beta variant favoring oligomerization in Alzheimer's-type dementia. Ann Neurol 2008;63:377–87.
93. Cairns NJ, Ikonomovic MD, Benzinger T, et al. Absence of Pittsburgh Compound B detection of cerebral amyloid beta in a patient with clinical, cognitive, and cerebrospinal fluid markers of Alzheimer disease: a case report. Arch Neurol 2009;66:1557–62.
94. Ikonomovic MD, Abrahamson EE, Price JC, et al. Early AD pathology in a [C-11] PiB-negative case: a PiB-amyloid imaging, biochemical, and immunohisto-chemical study. Acta Neuropathol 2012;123:433–47.
95. Aizenstein HJ, Nebes RD, Saxton JA, et al. Frequent amyloid deposition without significant cognitive impairment among the elderly. Arch Neurol 2008;65: 1509–17.
96. Mormino EC, Kluth JT, Madison CM, et al. Episodic memory loss is related to hippocampal-mediated beta-amyloid deposition in elderly subjects. Brain 2009;132:1310–23.
97. Reiman EM, Chen K, Liu X, et al. Fibrillar amyloid-beta burden in cognitively normal people at 3 levels of genetic risk for Alzheimer's disease. Proc Natl Acad Sci U S A 2009;106:6820–5.
98. Rowe CC, Ellis KA, Rimajova M, et al. Amyloid imaging results from the Australian Imaging, Biomarkers and Lifestyle (AIBL) study of aging. Neurobiol Aging 2010;31:1275–83.
99. Davies L, Wolska B, Hilbich C, et al. A4 amyloid protein deposition and the diagnosis of Alzheimer's disease: prevalence in aged brains determined by

immunocytochemistry compared with conventional neuropathologic techniques. Neurology 1988;38:1688–93.

100. Morris JC, Price AL. Pathologic correlates of nondemented aging, mild cognitive impairment, and early-stage Alzheimer's disease. J Mol Neurosci 2001;17:101–18.

101. Pike KE, Ellis KA, Villemagne VL, et al. Cognition and beta-amyloid in preclinical Alzheimer's disease: Data from the AIBL study. Neuropsychologia 2011;49: 2384–90.

102. Sperling RA, Johnson KA, Doraiswamy PM, et al. Amyloid deposition detected with florbetapir F 18 ((18)F-AV-45) is related to lower episodic memory performance in clinically normal older individuals. Neurobiol Aging 2013;34:822–31.

103. Winblad B, Palmer K, Kivipelto M, et al. Mild cognitive impairment—beyond controversies, towards a consensus: report of the International Working Group on Mild Cognitive Impairment. J Intern Med 2004;256:240–6.

104. Petersen RC, Smith GE, Ivnik RJ, et al. Apolipoprotein E status as a predictor of the development of Alzheimer's disease in memory-impaired individuals. JAMA 1995;273:1274–8.

105. Forsberg A, Engler H, Almkvist O, et al. PET imaging of amyloid deposition in patients with mild cognitive impairment. Neurobiol Aging 2008;29:1456–65.

106. Kemppainen NM, Aalto S, Wilson IA, et al. PET amyloid ligand [11C]PIB uptake is increased in mild cognitive impairment. Neurology 2007;68:1603–6.

107. Lowe VJ, Kemp BJ, Jack CR Jr, et al. Comparison of 18F-FDG and PiB PET in cognitive impairment. J Nucl Med 2009;50:878–86.

108. Pike KE, Savage G, Villemagne VL, et al. Beta-amyloid imaging and memory in non-demented individuals: evidence for preclinical Alzheimer's disease. Brain 2007;130:2837–44.

109. Rentz DM, Locascio JJ, Becker JA, et al. Cognition, reserve, and amyloid deposition in normal aging. Ann Neurol 2010;67:353–64.

110. Roe CM, Mintun MA, D'Angelo G, et al. Alzheimer disease and cognitive reserve: variation of education effect with carbon 11-labeled Pittsburgh Compound B uptake. Arch Neurol 2008;65:1467–71.

111. Cohen AD, Price JC, Weissfeld LA, et al. Basal cerebral metabolism may modulate the cognitive effects of Abeta in mild cognitive impairment: an example of brain reserve. J Neurosci 2009;29:14770–8.

112. Furst AJ, Rabinovici GD, Rostomian AH, et al. Cognition, glucose metabolism and amyloid burden in Alzheimer's disease. Neurobiol Aging 2012;33:215–25.

113. Resnick SM, Sojkova J, Zhou Y, et al. Longitudinal cognitive decline is associated with fibrillar amyloid-beta measured by [11C]PiB. Neurology 2010;74:807–15.

114. Villemagne VL, Pike KE, Darby D, et al. Aβ deposits in older non-demented individuals with cognitive decline are indicative of preclinical Alzheimer's disease. Neuropsychologia 2008;46:1688–97.

115. Doraiswamy PM, Sperling RA, Coleman RE, et al. Amyloid-beta assessed by florbetapir F 18 PET and 18-month cognitive decline: a multicenter study. Neurology 2012;79:1636–44.

116. Morris JC, Roe CM, Grant EA, et al. Pittsburgh Compound B imaging and prediction of progression from cognitive normality to symptomatic Alzheimer disease. Arch Neurol 2009;66:1469–75.

117. Nordberg A, Carter SF, Rinne J, et al. A European multicentre PET study of fibrillar amyloid in Alzheimer's disease. Eur J Nucl Med Mol Imaging 2012. http://dx.doi.org/10.1007/s00259-012-2237-2.

118. Okello A, Koivunen J, Edison P, et al. Conversion of amyloid positive and negative MCI to AD over 3 years: an 11C-PIB PET study. Neurology 2009;73:754–60.

119. Wolk DA, Price JC, Saxton JA, et al. Amyloid imaging in mild cognitive impairment subtypes. Ann Neurol 2009;65:557–68.

120. Sperling RA, Jack CR Jr, Aisen PS. Testing the right target and right drug at the right stage. Sci Transl Med 2011;3:111cm133.

121. Chetelat G, Villemagne VL, Pike KE, et al. Larger temporal volume in elderly with high versus low beta-amyloid deposition. Brain 2010;133:3349–58.

122. Tucker AM, Stern Y. Cognitive reserve in aging. Curr Alzheimer Res 2011;8: 354–60.

123. Ng S, Villemagne VL, Berlangieri S, et al. Visual assessment versus quantitative assessment of 11C-PIB PET and 18F-FDG PET for detection of Alzheimer's disease. J Nucl Med 2007;48:547–52.

124. Rabinovici GD, Rosen HJ, Alkalay A, et al. Amyloid vs FDG-PET in the differential diagnosis of AD and FTLD. Neurology 2011;77:2034–42.

125. DeKosky ST, Ikonomovic MD, Styren SD, et al. Upregulation of choline acetyltransferase activity in hippocampus and frontal cortex of elderly subjects with mild cognitive impairment. Ann Neurol 2002;51:145–55.

126. Ikonomovic MD, Abrahamson EE, Isanski BA, et al. Superior frontal cortex cholinergic axon density in mild cognitive impairment and early Alzheimer disease. Arch Neurol 2007;64:1312–7.

127. Herholz K. FDG PET and differential diagnosis of dementia. Alzheimer Dis Assoc Disord 1995;9:6–16.

128. Ikonomovic MD, Klunk WE, Abrahamson EE, et al. Precuneus amyloid burden is associated with reduced cholinergic activity in Alzheimer disease. Neurology 2011;77:39–47.

129. Blennow K, Zetterberg H, Minthon L, et al. Longitudinal stability of CSF biomarkers in Alzheimer's disease. Neurosci Lett 2007;419:18–22.

130. de Leon MJ, Mosconi L, Blennow K, et al. Imaging and CSF studies in the preclinical diagnosis of Alzheimer's disease. Ann N Y Acad Sci 2007;1097: 114–45.

131. Hansson O, Zetterberg H, Buchhave P, et al. Prediction of Alzheimer's disease using the CSF Abeta42/Abeta40 ratio in patients with mild cognitive impairment. Dement Geriatr Cogn Disord 2007;23:316–20.

132. Mattsson N, Andreasson U, Persson S, et al. The Alzheimer's Association external quality control program for cerebrospinal fluid biomarkers. Alzheimers Dement 2011;7:386–395.e6.

133. Forsberg A, Almkvist O, Engler H, et al. High PIB retention in Alzheimer's disease is an early event with complex relationship with CSF biomarkers and functional parameters. Curr Alzheimer Res 2010;7:56–66.

134. Tolboom N, van der Flier WM, Yaqub M, et al. Relationship of cerebrospinal fluid markers to 11C-PiB and 18F-FDDNP binding. J Nucl Med 2009;50: 1464–70.

135. Fagan AM, Mintun MA, Shah AR, et al. Cerebrospinal fluid tau and ptau(181) increase with cortical amyloid deposition in cognitively normal individuals: implications for future clinical trials of Alzheimer's disease. EMBO Mol Med 2009;1: 371–80.

136. Fagan AM, Roe CM, Xiong C, et al. Cerebrospinal fluid tau/beta-amyloid(42) ratio as a prediction of cognitive decline in nondemented older adults. Arch Neurol 2007;64:343–9.

137. Grimmer T, Riemenschneider M, Forstl H, et al. Beta amyloid in Alzheimer's disease: increased deposition in brain is reflected in reduced concentration in cerebrospinal fluid. Biol Psychiatry 2009;65:927–34.

138. Koivunen J, Pirttila T, Kemppainen N, et al. PET Amyloid Ligand [C]PIB Uptake and Cerebrospinal Fluid beta-Amyloid in Mild Cognitive Impairment. Dement Geriatr Cogn Disord 2008;26:378–83.

139. Apostolova LG, Hwang KS, Andrawis JP, et al. 3D PIB and CSF biomarker associations with hippocampal atrophy in ADNI subjects. Neurobiol Aging 2010;31: 1284–303.

140. Shaw LM, Korecka M, Clark CM, et al. Biomarkers of neurodegeneration for diagnosis and monitoring therapeutics. Nat Rev Drug Discov 2007;6:295–303.

141. Frisoni GB, Fox NC, Jack CR Jr, et al. The clinical use of structural MRI in Alzheimer disease. Nat Rev Neurol 2010;6:67–77.

142. Archer HA, Edison P, Brooks DJ, et al. Amyloid load and cerebral atrophy in Alzheimer's disease: an 11C-PIB positron emission tomography study. Ann Neurol 2006;60:145–7.

143. Becker JA, Hedden T, Carmasin J, et al. Amyloid-beta associated cortical thinning in clinically normal elderly. Ann Neurol 2011;69:1032–42.

144. Bourgeat P, Chetelat G, Villemagne VL, et al. Beta-amyloid burden in the temporal neocortex is related to hippocampal atrophy in elderly subjects without dementia. Neurology 2010;74:121–7.

145. Chetelat G, Villemagne VL, Bourgeat P, et al. Relationship between atrophy and beta-amyloid deposition in Alzheimer disease. Ann Neurol 2010;67:317–24.

146. Tosun D, Schuff N, Mathis CA, et al. Spatial patterns of brain amyloid-beta burden and atrophy rate associations in mild cognitive impairment. Brain 2011;134:1077–88.

147. Forster S, Grimmer T, Miederer I, et al. Regional expansion of hypometabolism in Alzheimer's disease follows amyloid deposition with temporal delay. Biol Psychiatry 2012;71:792–7.

148. Chetelat G, Villemagne VL, Villain N, et al. Accelerated cortical atrophy in cognitively normal elderly with high beta-amyloid deposition. Neurology 2012;78: 477–84.

149. Farrer LA, Cupples LA, Haines JL, et al. Effects of age, sex, and ethnicity on the association between apolipoprotein E genotype and Alzheimer disease. A meta-analysis. APOE and Alzheimer Disease Meta Analysis Consortium. JAMA 1997; 278:1349–56.

150. Berg L, McKeel DW Jr, Miller JP, et al. Clinicopathologic studies in cognitively healthy aging and Alzheimer's disease: relation of histologic markers to dementia severity, age, sex, and apolipoprotein E genotype. Arch Neurol 1998;55:326–35.

151. Rabinovici GD, Furst AJ, Alkalay A, et al. Increased metabolic vulnerability in early-onset Alzheimer's disease is not related to amyloid burden. Brain 2010; 133:512–28.

152. Bateman RJ, Xiong C, Benzinger TL, et al. Clinical and biomarker changes in dominantly inherited Alzheimer's disease. N Engl J Med 2012;367:795–804.

153. Landt J, D'Abrera JC, Holland AJ, et al. Using positron emission tomography and Carbon 11-labeled Pittsburgh Compound B to image Brain Fibrillar beta-amyloid in adults with down syndrome: safety, acceptability, and feasibility. Arch Neurol 2011;68:890–6.

154. Villemagne VL, Pike K, Pejoska S, et al. 11C-PiB PET ABri imaging in Worster-Drought syndrome (familial British dementia): a case report. J Alzheimers Dis 2010;19:423–8.

155. Gomperts SN, Rentz DM, Moran E, et al. Imaging amyloid deposition in Lewy body diseases. Neurology 2008;71:903–10.

156. Maetzler W, Liepelt I, Reimold M, et al. Cortical PIB binding in Lewy body disease is associated with Alzheimer-like characteristics. Neurobiol Dis 2009; 34:107–12.

157. Johnson KA, Gregas M, Becker JA, et al. Imaging of amyloid burden and distribution in cerebral amyloid angiopathy. Ann Neurol 2007;62:229–34.

158. Drzezga A, Grimmer T, Henriksen G, et al. Imaging of amyloid plaques and cerebral glucose metabolism in semantic dementia and Alzheimer's disease. Neuroimage 2008;39:619–33.

159. Engler H, Santillo AF, Wang SX, et al. In vivo amyloid imaging with PET in frontotemporal dementia. Eur J Nucl Med Mol Imaging 2008;35:100–6.

160. Pletnikova O, West N, Lee MK, et al. Abeta deposition is associated with enhanced cortical a-synuclein lesions in Lewy body diseases. Neurobiol Aging 2005;26:1183–92.

161. Masliah E, Rockenstein E, Veinbergs I, et al. Beta-amyloid peptides enhance alpha-synuclein accumulation and neuronal deficits in a transgenic mouse model linking Alzheimer's disease and Parkinson's disease. Proc Natl Acad Sci U S A 2001;98:12245–50.

162. Halliday G, Hely M, Reid W, et al. The progression of pathology in longitudinally followed patients with Parkinson's disease. Acta Neuropathol 2008;115:409–15.

163. Rabinovici GD, Miller BL. Frontotemporal lobar degeneration: epidemiology, pathophysiology, diagnosis and management. CNS Drugs 2010;24:375–98.

164. Leyton CE, Villemagne VL, Savage S, et al. Subtypes of progressive aphasia: application of the international consensus criteria and validation using {beta}-amyloid imaging. Brain 2011;134:3030–43.

165. Rabinovici GD, Jagust WJ, Furst AJ, et al. Abeta amyloid and glucose metabolism in three variants of primary progressive aphasia. Ann Neurol 2008;64:388–401.

Relevance of Magnetic Resonance Imaging for Early Detection and Diagnosis of Alzheimer Disease

Stefan J. Teipel, MD[a,b,*], Michel Grothe, PhD[b], Simone Lista, PhD[c],
Nicola Toschi, PhD[d], Francesco G. Garaci, PhD[e,f],
Harald Hampel, MD[c]

KEYWORDS

- Alzheimer disease • Preclinical diagnosis • Magnetic resonance imaging
- Functional magnetic resonance imaging • Diffusion tensor imaging
- Diffusion spectrum imaging • Multimodal imaging • Prediction

KEY POINTS

- Hippocampus volumetry currently is the best-established imaging biomarker for Alzheimer disease (AD).
- Imaging markers need further validation in respect of the underlying neurobiological substrate and potential confounds such as vascular disease, inflammation, hydrocephalus, and alcoholism, and clinical outcomes such as cognition, but also as regards demographic and socioeconomic outcomes such as mortality and institutionalization.
- More advanced imaging protocols, including diffusion tensor imaging, diffusion spectrum imaging, and functional magnetic resonance imaging (MRI), are presently being used in monocenter and first multicenter studies.
- From a neurobiological point of view, the main determinants of cognitive impairment in AD are the density of synapses and neurons in distributed cortical and subcortical networks.
- MRI-based measures of regional gray matter volume and associated multivariate analysis techniques of regional interactions of gray matter densities provide insight into the onset and temporal dynamics of cortical atrophy as a close proxy for regional neuronal loss and as basis of functional impairment in specific neuronal networks.

Funding: H.H. was supported by the Katharina-Hardt-Foundation, Bad Homburg, Germany. S.J.T. was supported by the Department AGIS of the University of Rostock.
[a] University Medicine Rostock, Rostock, Germany; [b] DZNE, German Center for Neurodegenerative Diseases, Rostock, Germany; [c] Department of Psychiatry, Goethe University, Frankfurt, Germany; [d] Medical Physics Section, Faculty of Medicine, University of Rome "Tor Vergata" (Via Montpellier 1 - 00133 Rome), Rome, Italy; [e] Department of Diagnostic Imaging and Interventional Radiology, University of Rome "Tor Vergata", Rome, Italy; [f] Institute for Research and Medical Care IRCCS San Raffaele (Via della Pisana 235), Rome, Italy
* Corresponding author.
E-mail address: stefan.teipel@med.uni-rostock.de

Med Clin N Am 97 (2013) 399–424
http://dx.doi.org/10.1016/j.mcna.2012.12.013
0025-7125/13/$ – see front matter © 2013 Elsevier Inc. All rights reserved.

INTRODUCTION

Alzheimer disease (AD) is the most common cause of dementia in the elderly. Autopsy case series on the sequential accumulation of neurofibrillary bundles and amyloid plaques, as well as on the progression of neuronal loss through the cerebral cortex, suggest that AD is a system-specific brain disease that affects discrete neuronal systems in a fairly consistent temporospatial pattern while other brain regions are widely spared or only affected in late stages of the disease.[1,2] The system specificity of pathologic events in AD and the preclinical onset of these changes have fueled the definition of new diagnostic criteria for preclinical and predementia AD that incorporate neuroimaging markers and biomarkers to define the presence of disease.[3–5]

According to current diagnostic criteria the diagnosis of AD is based on clinical history, psychiatric and neurologic examination, neuropsychological testing, and supportive measures including structural imaging and blood tests to exclude other causes of dementia.[6] The inclusion of biomarkers from structural, functional, and molecular imaging in the revised diagnostic criteria aims both to improve specificity for the diagnosis of AD dementia[7] and to reach a diagnosis of AD before the onset of manifest dementia. These criteria are primarily intended for use in research settings but may also affect the clinical diagnosis of early stages of AD in the future.

Following the amyloid cascade hypothesis,[8] molecular lesions of neurotoxic amyloid accumulation in the cerebral cortex are the first event of a pathologic cascade involving synaptic dysfunction, axonal degeneration and, finally, neuronal loss. Neuronal loss can be detected using measures of brain atrophy in structural magnetic resonance imaging (MRI),[9] and already affects specific brain regions years before the onset of clinical dementia.[10] A high-resolution structural MRI scan on a 1.5- or 3-T MRI scanner requires only 5 to 10 minutes of acquisition time. The technique is widely available, and some analysis methods have already been established since the early 1990s. Therefore, structural MRI has become a key imaging biomarker for prodromal or predementia AD.

In the following sections this article discusses how structural MRI findings reflect the systematic nature of AD progression through the brain, confirming and extending the initial findings by Braak and Braak[1] on the temporospatial patterns of system-specific brain changes associated with AD, and how these changes can be used to improve diagnostic accuracy in early AD. The review proceeds from the most easily accessible approaches of visual rating, through manual volumetry, to automated data-driven analyses involving univariate or multivariate statistics.

Several criteria have been postulated for the use of biological measures as diagnostic markers or potential end points to assess treatment effects: (1) applicability (ie, the test should be noninvasive, widely available, and pose low patient burden), (2) reliability, both within one center (test-retest reliability) and across centers, and (3) validity in respect to underlying pathology and clinical outcomes.[11] Structural MRI is widely applicable and poses, in general, relatively low patient burden. The reliability of volumetric measures obtained from repeated MRI scans is generally high.[12,13] Less is known about the variability of volumetric measures obtained from different MRI scanners. The variability of manual and automated volumetric measures across 12 different MRI scanners was below 5% in one study,[14] for manual volumetric measurement of the hippocampus only 3.5%, despite a rather liberal acquisition protocol across centers. This variation is in the range of accuracy of manual or automated segmentation protocols tested against simple or complex phantoms in a single-center approach,[13] suggesting that multicenter variability, once minimal criteria for scanner quality are met by the participating centers, will not limit the application of structural MRI in clinical trials. Clinical validity in terms of prediction of functional outcomes in predementia stages was a major focus of structural imaging research in the last years. Autopsy diagnosis as gold standard end point has been applied only in few studies so far, and a small number of analysis approaches have been assessed with respect to pathologic validity. Clinicopathologic comparison studies have shown that hippocampus volume obtained antemortem accounted for at least 50% of variability in neuron numbers determined during autopsy.[15] The amount of variation explained by MRI-based hippocampus volumetry was above 90% when MRI scans had been obtained post mortem.[9] Thus, hippocampus volumetry can be considered as an in vivo surrogate measure of hippocampal neuronal density. One should, however, be careful in simply interpolating these findings to in vivo measures of cortical atrophy. In 27 antemortem cognitively intact subjects, cortical thinning determined post mortem across age cohorts was not associated with regional neuron numbers and density, but was suggested to reflect changes in neuronal and dendritic architecture.[16] Therefore, the interpretation of imaging findings is always founded on some prior concept of underlying disease mechanisms.

THE DIAGNOSTIC USE OF MRI IN AD

The neurodegeneration in AD leads to a marked reduction of brain tissue, which on MRI scans primarily presents as signal loss in the medial temporal lobe (MTL) and widening of cerebrospinal fluid (CSF) spaces. At the end of the last century, increasing evidence from postmortem autopsy studies pointed to a temporospatial pattern of progressive AD pathology that manifests at first in the perirhinal and entorhinal cortices of the MTL and extends sequentially to include other allocortical regions followed by neocortical association areas of the temporal, parietal, and frontal lobes. Primary sensorimotor areas are relatively spared or affected only in highly advanced stages of the disease.[1] Based on these observations, a neuropathologic staging scheme of AD severity into 6 stages of cortical involvement was proposed. Of importance, this staging scheme predicted that the first stages of AD pathology, the "transentorhinal" stages I and II, correspond to clinically silent cases, whereas the "limbic" (III and IV) and "neocortical" (V and VI) stages are usually associated with incipient and fully developed AD dementia, respectively (**Fig. 1**). An overview on MRI markers is given in **Table 1**.

Visual Ratings

The simplest approach to determine regional changes of brain volumes is to use visual rating scales based on digital images or hard copies of a 3-dimensional MRI sequence.[17] These scales have a high accuracy in determining the extent of atrophy in cross-sectional studies relative to more labor-intensive manual volumetry of the hippocampus,[17–19] and reached an accuracy of about 89% in discriminating AD patients from controls in a small sample of subjects.[20] By contrast, the use of a visual rating scale to determine rates of atrophy over time only reached accuracy at chance level relative to volumetric measures, suggesting that this approach may not be useful as a secondary end point in clinical trials.[19] This finding illustrates that information on reliability of new markers cannot simply be interpolated from cross-sectional to longitudinal study designs.

Manual Volumetry

Given the prominence of MTL atrophy on MRI scans, which corresponds to postmortem evidence of earliest and most severe neurofibrillary degeneration in this

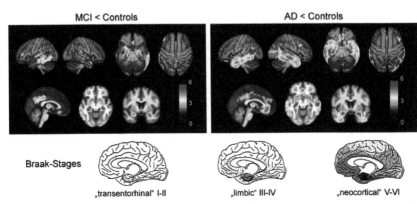

Fig. 1. Cortical atrophy in MRI and Braak staging. (*Upper row*) Voxel-wise maps of gray matter volume reductions in a group of subjects with mild cognitive impairment (MCI) (n = 69) and a group of AD patients (n = 28), respectively, compared with the same group of healthy age-matched controls (n = 95). Unpublished data; MRI images retrieved from publicly available database (www.oasis-brains.org). (*Lower row*) drawings of the Braak staging scheme of neurofibrillary pathology in AD. Note that voxel-wise pattern of gray matter atrophy in MCI and AD resemble the "limbic" and "neocortical" stages of neurofibrillary degeneration, respectively, as outlined by Braak and Braak. (*Adapted from* Braak H, Braak E. Staging of Alzheimer's disease-related neurofibrillary changes. Neurobiol Aging 1995;16(3):271–8; with permission from granted by Karger AG, Basel.)

region, first attempts to quantify AD-related atrophy on in vivo MRI scans focused on volumetric measurements of MTL structures, most notably the hippocampus.[21,22] Manually measured hippocampus volumes in patients with AD dementia showed a consistent reduction of up to 40% compared with healthy controls of the same age, allowing for highly accurate group separations based on the MRI scan only. Hippocampal volume as measured by MRI scans post mortem or in end stages of disease was further shown to account for a high proportion of 50% to 80% of variance in measures of neuronal loss and neurofibrillary abnormality at autopsy.[9,23] Whereas subregions of the MTL showed comparably high degrees of atrophy even in mild stages of AD,[24,25] neocortical involvement was more consistently detected in advanced stages of AD dementia, and showed a pattern of declining atrophy severity from temporal over parietal to frontal and occipital lobes.[26,27]

The Braak staging scheme of progressive neurofibrillary degeneration predicts earliest structural changes to precede the onset of dementia by several years, and thus AD-typical atrophy patterns on MRI should also be detectable in asymptomatic or very mildly impaired subjects at high risk of developing AD. One of those risk groups is given by subjects with a diagnosis of amnestic mild cognitive impairment (MCI), which is defined as a relatively isolated memory impairment that is greater as what is expected by age alone, but is not severe enough to interfere with activities of daily living and does not suffice for a diagnosis of dementia.[28] Patients diagnosed with MCI exhibit an increased risk for developing AD with incidence rates of 10% to 15% per year, compared with 1% to 2% per year for healthy unimpaired subjects of the same age. The syndrome is seen as a boundary or transitional stage between normal aging and dementia, and often reflects prodromal AD pathology.[29] When comparing temporal lobe volumes between healthy elderly subjects, individuals with a diagnosis of MCI, and AD patients, a significant reduction of hippocampus volume was detectable in the MCI (−14%) and the AD groups (−22%), but atrophy of the temporal neocortex was found only in the AD group.[30] Of interest is that in a clinical follow-up study on subjects with MCI, neocortical temporal lobe volume was already reduced in those subjects who later declined to AD, which significantly distinguished them from the MCI subjects who remained stable.[31]

In terms of diagnostic accuracies, volumes of the hippocampus and the entorhinal cortex can separate AD patients and MCI subjects from healthy controls, with accuracies ranging from 70% for early stages of MCI to complete group separation for advanced stages of AD dementia.[21,25,32] Furthermore, volumes of both hippocampus and entorhinal cortex predict future conversion to AD in individuals with MCI at accuracies around 80% to 85%, whereas the predictive value of entorhinal cortex volume seems to be slightly superior over hippocampus volume.[33–35] An important issue is the added value of volumetric measurements over other predictors, such as age and neuropsychological performance. In 139 MCI subjects followed over an average interval of 5 years, age, Mini Mental State Examination score, delayed recall, and digit symbol test performance predicted conversion to AD with almost 80% accuracy. Adding volumes of hippocampus and entorhinal cortex to the prediction model increased accuracy to 87%.[36] Although the diagnostic value of neuropsychological performance may be slightly overestimated as it is at least an indirect criterion to define conversion to dementia, these data indicate that the added value of MTL volumes may be significant, but clinically moderate.

Considering the diagnostic use of entorhinal cortex volume versus hippocampus volume, cross-sectional studies suggest that entorhinal cortex volumetry is unlikely to provide any additional benefit over hippocampus volume in identifying patients with AD dementia in comparison with controls[25,37–39]; however, at the MCI stage it may improve prognostic efficiency by a few percent compared with hippocampal volumetry,[32,38] although one multicenter study suggests no additional benefit.[40]

Especially informative for the study of earliest structural changes in the course of AD is MRI data of longitudinally followed elderly who were completely asymptomatic at the time of the MRI scan and later developed cognitive impairments leading to diagnoses of MCI or AD. Using such data, a few studies were able to show that volumetric reduction of the anterior MTL, including the hippocampus, the amygdala, and the entorhinal cortex, precedes the onset of cognitive deterioration by several years.[41–43] Thus, volumes of the amygdala and the hippocampus in clinically declining subjects were found to be on average 5% smaller than in stable controls as early as 6 years before the diagnosis of dementia was made. An individual risk prediction, however, is not possible based on these atrophy measures in cognitively healthy subjects.

Results on MTL volumetry are still heterogeneous, not the least because of different measurement protocols with different anatomic criteria used to define and outline the hippocampus. At present, a combined effort of the European Alzheimer's Disease Consortium (EADC) and the Alzheimer's Disease Neuroimaging Initiative (ADNI) is under way to harmonize protocols for the manual tracing of the hippocampus with the goal of developing and validating a unified standard protocol.[44] This protocol would eventually serve as gold-standard reference for the training of automated hippocampus volumetry.

Hippocampus Subfields

The wide availability of high-field MRI at 3 T and the increasing availability of ultrahigh-field MRI at 7 T rendered subfield measurements of the hippocampus a feasible diagnostic approach in selected samples. Pathologic evidence suggests a selective vulnerability of hippocampal subfields in AD.[10] Both manual volumetric and atlas-based automated measurements have been used to determine volumes of CA1 to CA4, dentate gyrus, and subiculum. The manual methods are extremely time

Table 1
Structural MRI markers for Alzheimer disease (AD)

Marker	Diagnostic Use	Longitudinal Marker	Comments
Visual rating of hippocampus volume	High correlation with hippocampus volume ($R^2 \sim 0.9$, diagnostic accuracy for AD vs controls between 80% and 90%,[19,20] prediction of AD in MCI not assessed. Reductions of hippocampus and adjacent MTL areas in preclinical stages, but no individual risk prediction	Detection of change at chance level[19]	Useful for diagnostic evaluation at baseline,[19,20] no use for follow-up. So far, no preclinical prediction in asymptomatic subjects for individual cases
Manual volumetry of hippocampus	Diagnostic accuracy for AD vs controls between 80% and 90%,[189] prediction of AD in MCI with 70%–80% accuracy[190]	Rates of atrophy about 4.7% per annum in AD compared with 0.9%–1.4% in healthy controls[191,192]	Already used in clinical trials as secondary end point; multicenter variability of longitudinal changes needs to be assessed
Automated volumetry of hippocampus	High correlation with manual volumetry ($R^2 > 0.8$).[78] Group discrimination AD vs controls 83%, MCI vs controls 73% (post hoc probability only).[56] 88% accuracy for the discrimination of MCI converters from stable MCI subjects[45,58]	Rate of atrophy predicts subsequent cognitive decline in nondemented elderly with about 80% accuracy.[193] Baseline volume correlates with subsequent cognitive decline in MCI[194]	First data from large multicenter studies suggest stable performance for diagnostic and predictive accuracy
Manual and automated hippocampus subfield measurements	In small sample studies, diagnostic accuracy of subfield measurements was superior to total hippocampus volume to discriminate MCI from healthy controls.[46,195,196] One study shows high predictive accuracy of hippocampus shape in preclinical subjects, but requires further confirmation[51]	Only little assessed in this respect so far	Approach that may prove useful in the context of clinical trials for risk stratification; no clinical application to date because of complexity of method and time-consuming delineation (manual approaches). Very limited data on predictive accuracy in preclinical and predementia stages[51]

Manual volumetry of entorhinal cortex	No additional benefit in identifying patients with manifest AD. Accuracy of prediction of AD in MCI increased by a few percent compared with hippocampus volumetry in monocenter studies,[38,197,198] no additional use in first multicenter studies[40]	Rates of ERC atrophy 5-times greater in AD than in controls,[199] but only applied in small-scale monocenter studies so far	Diagnostic use for prognosis of AD in MCI seems to be superior to hippocampus; use as secondary end point in RCT seems not superior to hippocampus considering the laborious methodology
Automated measurement of whole brain volume	Diagnostic use only for the rate of change, not the baseline volume, but would require second scan after 1 y before diagnosis can be supported	Atrophy rate of 2.5% per year in AD patients compared with 0.4%–0.9% in healthy controls.[200,201] Multicenter stability has not systematically been assessed	Already secondary end point in clinical trials, but only limited heuristic value because of global nature of the measurement
Voxel-based morphometry	Characteristic pattern of brain atrophy in AD and MCI, but lacks an established statistical model to determine individual risk for a single subject. Combining VBM with ROIs yields 78% sensitivity and 75% specificity in predicting MCI in healthy subjects,[202] but only post hoc probability	Accelerated rates of regional gray matter atrophy in patients with MCI who later converted to AD,[74] but no established model for effect size estimation of outcome	The combination of VBM with an ROI approach allows diagnostic use, but abandons the advantage of mapping changes across the entire brain[40]
Deformation-based morphometry	Statistical models for individual risk prediction have been proposed: predicts AD in MCI with 80%–90% accuracy,[177,178] discriminates between MCI and controls with 90% accuracy.[179]	Characteristic spread of atrophy through the brain in AD.[203] No data from intervention studies, no established statistical model for evaluation of intervention effects	Allows individual risk prediction based on information on atrophy pattern across the entire brain. Awaits confirmation in larger multicenter and longitudinal studies
Cortical thickness measurement	90% accuracy in the discrimination between AD patients and controls.[60] Reaches effect sizes similar to manual hippocampus volumetry when predicting AD in MCI[40]	Provides an easily accessible end point such as an average rate of 0.18 mm atrophy per year in AD[204]	Promising end point in clinical trials, as it offers a direct assessment of effect sizes expressed in a meaningful metric

Abbreviations: ERC, entorhinal cortex; MCI, mild cognitive impairment; MTL, medial temporal lobe; RCT, randomized controlled trial; ROI, region of interest; VBM, voxel-based morphometry.

consuming, with several hours of tracing per scan. At the same time they are based on the direct identification of anatomic boundaries, and therefore serve as gold standard to assess the performance of automated methods.

Using total hippocampus volume as predictor for future conversion from MCI to AD, the false-negative rate is still 30%.[45] In studies on a small number of subjects, the assessment of CA1 and CA2 using manual delineation[46] and CA2 to CA3 using automated delineation[47] was more accurate than total hippocampus volume in discriminating MCI subjects from controls. Obviously the technique of analysis matters, and thus subfields that were found most atrophic differ slightly between surface mapping, automated atlas-based labeling, and manual measurement approaches. Sequences at 7 T provide access to even finer substructures of the hippocampus, but the clinical relevance of these measures is still unclear.[48]

A purely data-driven approach to determine within-hippocampus differences with aging or disease is hippocampus shape analysis. Based on high parametric deformation algorithms, shape models of the hippocampus can automatically be determined. Data-reducing approaches, such as principal component analysis, allow extraction of characteristic parameters from these individual shape models that can be compared between diagnostic groups. In a small-scale study of 18 AD patients and 26 controls, this approach yielded 67% sensitivity and 85% specificity in the discrimination between AD patients and controls.[49] A multivariate analysis based on support vector machine classification of automatically extracted hippocampus shape features yielded discrimination accuracy between AD patients and controls of 94%, and accuracy between MCI subjects and controls of 83%.[50] In a study on 139 subjects who were free of cognitive impairment at baseline and were followed over 10 years, hippocampal shape analysis revealed a cluster at the ventromedial head of the right hippocampus that predicted conversion to AD with about 90% accuracy.[51] This interesting result clearly requires further replication, as an overfitting of the data cannot always be excluded with these complex models.

Automated Region-Driven Methods

Manual volumetric methods are associated with several drawbacks that limit their utility for the assessment of brain atrophy in neurodegenerative diseases. Most notably, manual delineation of regions of interest (ROIs) is rater dependent, relatively labor intensive, and limited to brain structures that provide clearly delineable borders defined by anatomic landmarks. Since the beginning of this century, automated methods have been under development to determine regionally specific changes in brain structure using hypothesis-driven and rater-independent approaches.[52,53]

Hypothesis-driven automated approaches focus on selected brain regions, such as the hippocampus, the cholinergic basal forebrain, or hippocampus subfields (see earlier discussion). Automated segmentations of the hippocampus exhibit high anatomic accuracy when compared with manual delineations[54,55] and provide comparable diagnostic power.[56,57] When tested for their diagnostic potential in large multicenter data sets, such as provided by the ADNI, automatically segmented volumes of the hippocampus achieve accuracies of around 70% and 80% for separating MCI subjects and AD patients, respectively, from healthy controls, and predict conversion to dementia in MCI subjects with 88% accuracy.[45,58]

However, diagnostic models based on single volumes do not account for the AD-typical pattern of progressive atrophy that spreads from the MTL to the temporoparietal neocortex early in the course of the disease. Modern image-processing software allows the automated parcellation of the brain in neuroanatomic ROIs that can then be tested separately and in combination for their diagnostic potential using logistic regression or discriminant analysis. Using such an approach, it could be shown in a multicenter setting that a combined structural marker of the hippocampus, the entorhinal cortex, and the temporoparietal junction could increase diagnostic accuracy for the separation of MCI from controls to 90%.[59] Optimal combinations of automatically extracted regional markers for distinguishing between AD patients and controls could even yield complete group separations.[59,60] Accordingly, composite markers that combined AD-typical regional measures, including the MTL, temporoparietal association areas, and medial parietal regions, showed promising accuracies of around 75% for the prediction of imminent conversion to AD in multicenter data of subjects with MCI.[61,62]

Automated Data-Driven Methods

For purely data-driven analyses, the most commonly used automated morphometry approach is voxel-based morphometry (VBM). In its original implementation the method is based on a low-dimensional spatial transformation of brain scans into a common reference space to control for global differences in brain size and shape. After segmentation of the scans into brain tissue and CSF spaces, remaining local differences in gray matter volumes, which are not modeled by the global spatial normalization, are the parameters of interest that drive a voxel-based univariate statistic. This approach has been criticized because the concept of global versus regional effects cannot be operationalized, and modeled effects will depend on the characteristics of the normalization algorithm. Furthermore, the accuracy of normalization may vary with neurobiological differences, and thus effects in VBM may be driven by group differences in normalization accuracy rather than the neurobiological differences themselves.[63] These arguments are a matter of debate[64] and are still not finally resolved. From a pragmatic perspective, VBM has widely been used and results from these analyses have proved to be reproducible across different scanners and processing approaches,[14] and to spatially agree with effects from other imaging techniques and autopsy studies.[65] There is, however, still no validation of VBM in respect of the underlying neurobiological changes, not the least because the counting of neuron numbers, the most likely substrate of measures of atrophy in AD, is difficult to perform for neocortical regions. Therefore, reference values for neuron numbers in cortical regions of the human brain are lacking. The validity of VBM-based measurements of cortical atrophy with respect to potential clinical outcomes such as memory performance has begun to be established recently.[66,67] Combined with results from other neurodegenerative dementias,[68,69] these data suggest that VBM reveals a pattern of brain atrophy whose relation to specific cognitive impairments is consistent with a priori models of the representation of cognitive function in cortical and subcortical neuronal networks in the human brain.

When applied to demented AD patients, VBM analyses demonstrate the expected pattern of global cortical atrophy that is most pronounced in medial and lateral temporoparietal cortices, with a relative sparing of the sensorimotor cortex, the occipital pole, and the cerebellum.[70,71] The spatial pattern of progressive neuropathology in AD as suggested by the postmortem autopsy studies was impressively demonstrated using VBM and serial MRI of MCI subjects who progressed to AD.[72] Hence, early atrophic changes in subjects with MCI, approximately 3 years before the clinical diagnosis of AD, were found to be confined to the MTL. At a later stage, but still with the diagnosis of MCI, atrophy had spread to include lateral temporal and temporoparietal association areas of the neocortex. At the time the diagnosis of AD was made, atrophy had become more severe and widespread and by then also involved areas of the prefrontal cortex, probably reflecting neurofibrillary-tangle abnormality of the neocortical Braak stages V and VI.[65] Accordingly, cross-sectional VBM studies on MCI consistently demonstrate atrophy of the MTL, whereas the degree of involvement of areas of neocortical association varies across studies, probably attributable to the heterogeneity of MCI as a transitional state between normal aging and AD.[73] Thus, MCI subjects with an imminent conversion to AD dementia show greater reductions in MTL volume but especially greater atrophy of the temporoparietal neocortex and the posterior cingulate/precuneus when compared with MCI subjects who remain stable during clinical follow-up.[40,74] Using serial MRI, it could be further shown that most of these regions not only showed lower volumes at baseline but also higher longitudinal rates of volume decline as MCI subjects progressed to a diagnosis of AD.[74,75]

Unbiased VBM studies could also complement manual volumetry findings of earliest structural changes in the (anterior) MTL in cognitively normal subjects who are destined to develop AD, by providing evidence for concomitant atrophy outside the MTL, including the basal forebrain[76] and the posterior cingulate/precuneus.[51] Analysis of serial MRI data over a follow-up of up to 10 consecutive years further revealed that age-related volume loss is apparent and widespread even in cognitively stable elderly, although the regional brain changes associated with a conversion to MCI differ significantly in location and magnitude from the pattern associated with normal brain aging.[77]

Advanced Image Analysis

Based on improvements in hardware and software resources, increasingly sophisticated computational methods for image processing and analysis are being developed that allow the automated segmentation and detailed subfield analysis of the hippocampus and other ROIs in large imaging datasets.[55,78,79] Modern computational methods demonstrate high anatomic accuracy of the segmented volumes when compared with manual volumetry techniques[54,80] and even allow for the detailed structural analysis of brain regions that are less amenable to manual delineation. The overarching principle behind the majority of these approaches is the use of high-dimensional image-deformation algorithms. Different to the classic VBM analysis, these deformation-based approaches use hundreds of thousands of nonlinear parameters to warp the individual brain images into the reference space, yielding a highly exact match to the template image and thereby eliminating spatial differences among the individual scans. The information on interindividual spatial variability then resides entirely in the deformation functions themselves, rendering the differentiation in global and regional effects obsolete. This approach opens the way for the high-resolution study of anatomic details by direct extraction of volumetric information from the individual deformation fields or by automated segmentation of the individual brains into structural or functional ROIs, based on inverse warping of detailed atlases in the template space.

While MRI research on structural brain atrophy in AD generally focuses on the MTL and neocortical regions, the involvement of subcortical nuclei across disease stages is less thoroughly explored. This fact is surprising given the prevalent neuropathologic evidence of selective involvement of specific subcortical areas, most notably the cholinergic nuclei of the basal forebrain,[81,82] and may be partly explained by technical issues associated with subcortical in vivo volumetry. The complex anatomy of the basal forebrain and the indistinguishability of cholinergic cells on normal MRI scans place important constraints on the in vivo structural analysis of cholinergic degeneration in AD.[83,84] However, the recent development of cytoarchitectonic maps of the cholinergic nuclei in MRI standard space, based on combined histology and postmortem MRI,[85,86] now renders the cholinergic basal forebrain amenable to in vivo volumetry by the use of advanced computational methods for automated regional volume extraction. Using such an approach the selective involvement of different cholinergic nuclei across disease stages could be studied in vivo. A progressive and differential decline in volume of the cholinergic subnuclei was found across the spectrum from normal aging over MCI to AD, resulting in severe atrophy of the nucleus basalis Meynert in patients with mild to moderate AD that was comparable in magnitude with atrophy of the hippocampus (**Fig. 2**).[87,88]

BEYOND STRUCTURAL MRI ACQUISITION AND ANALYSIS: RESEARCH PERSPECTIVES AND FUTURE CLINICAL APPLICATIONS

During the last decade, several advanced MR modalities have been applied to the study of AD and have widened the field for the design of potential markers that may aid in identifying individuals at risk of developing AD. Although such applications have been primarily targeted to research (as opposed to clinical) applications, the complementary information provided by multimodal MR imaging could eventually be integrated (eg, through machine-learning techniques) to aid in diagnosis, disease screening, and risk stratification.

Diffusion-Weighted Imaging, Gaussian and Non-Gaussian

Diffusion tensor imaging (DTI)[89] has been extremely successful in investigating white matter microarchitecture, connectivity, and integrity, and has been widely used in studies investigating AD and MCI.[90–92] Modern echo planar imaging (EPI) techniques[93]

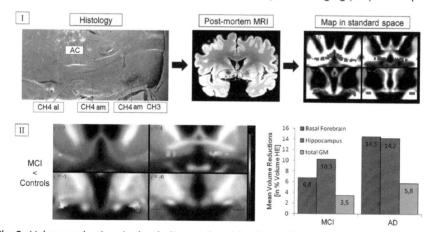

Fig. 2. Volume reductions in the cholinergic basal forebrain. (*I*) Generation of a cytoarchitectonic map of basal forebrain cholinergic nuclei in MRI standard space. Cholinergic cells are stained in histologic slices and cholinergic nuclei are manually transferred to a corresponding postmortem MRI, which is then automatically normalized into MRI standard space as defined by the Montreal Neurological Institute (MNI). Figures based on data published in Ref.[88] AC, anterior commissure; CH3, cholinergic cells corresponding to the horizontal limb of the diagonal band of Broca; CH4 am, CH4 al, cholinergic cells corresponding to the anterior medial and lateral parts of the nucleus basalis Meynert. (*II*) Left: voxel-wise reductions in gray matter volume within the basal forebrain region of interest in MCI subjects compared with healthy controls. Right: group means of extracted basal forebrain, hippocampus, and total gray matter (GM) volumes in groups of MCI subjects and AD patients plotted as percent volume reduction compared with a healthy elderly (HE) reference group. (*Data from* Bozzali M, Cherubini A. Diffusion tensor MRI to investigate dementias: a brief review. Magn Reson Imaging 2007;25(6):969–77.)

allow relatively rapid (4–9 minutes) whole-brain estimation of the apparent water diffusion tensor (DT) field, and DT-derived rotational invariants such as the single DT eigenvalues, mean diffusivity (MD) (the mean of DT eigenvalues), and fractional anisotropy (FA) (normalized variance of DT eigenvalues[94]) can aid in quantifying fiber integrity through ROI or voxel-based approaches.[91] In addition, DTI can provide information about architecture of white matter tracts, which is commonly quantified through deterministic and/or or probabilistic tractography approaches.[95] Several studies have revealed a decrease in FA (commonly accompanied by an increase in MD or in 1 or more eigenvalues) in AD and MCI.[96–98] This finding typically indicates unspecific bundle degeneration, and correlations between white matter integrity and disease severity have also been reported in AD,[99,100] suggesting that DTI measures may be used as indices of disease progression.[101] Although early (MCI stage) alterations in white matter have been detected within the parahippocampal gyrus, posterior cingulum, and splenium of the corpus callosum,[102–105] most DTI-based investigations of MCI and AD point to the uncinate fasciculus, the entire corpus callosum, and the cingulum tract as the most affected regions. Of note, a recent study that included both AD and MCI patients[106] found a circumscribed increase in FA in the MCI group. The interpretation of these findings was aided by the introduction of a third tensor invariant (tensor mode [MO]),[107] which is able to distinguish the "type" of anisotropy (planar, eg, in regions of crossing fibers, vs linear, in regions where a single coherent orientation dominates). In regions of increased FA, an accompanying increase in MO (which indicates a transition toward a more linear anisotropy) pointed toward the hypothesis of a selective degeneration of only 1 of 2 crossing fibers, in this case indicating a relative preservation of motor-related projection fibers crossing the association tracts of the superior longitudinal fasciculus in the early-stage MCI patients. Also, DTI appears to be able to detect progressive white matter degeneration in AD as it advances with aging. In agreement with the retrogenesis model (cortical regions that mature earliest in infancy tend to degenerate last in AD), white matter abnormalities seem to appear earliest in selected brain regions such as prefrontal cortex white matter, the inferior longitudinal fasciculus, and temporoparietal areas.[91,102,108,109] It should be noted that reproducibility and robustness play a prominent role in (comparatively noisy) DTI acquisitions, and a recent meta-analysis indicates high variability in both the anatomy of regions studied and DTI-derived metrics.[110] In this context, a recent European multicenter study[111] highlighted significant center-related effects in DTI-derived measures. Also, the simplistic model of a Gaussian propagator, which is at the base of DTI, may reach its limits in regions/voxels containing mixed tissue types and/or where 2 or more fiber bundles cross.[112] To this end more advanced protocols, such as diffusion spectrum imaging,[113] diffusional kurtosis imaging,[114–116] higher-order tensor models,[117] compartment models,[118,119] and anomalous diffusion,[120,121] have been developed to enhance their suitability in a clinical setting,[122] and have already been successfully used in augmenting information about tissue degeneration in several disorders including AD (**Fig. 3**).[123–126]

Functional Magnetic Resonance Imaging: Task-Based and Resting State

Neuronal activity can be studied noninvasively (albeit indirectly) through blood oxygenation level dependent (BOLD) functional MRI (fMRI), and several fMRI studies have been able to detect functional alterations that precede AD symptoms and quantifiable AD-related structural neurodegeneration.[127–129] Standard task-based fMRI protocols have used episodic memory tasks in studying memory-related activation in the hippocampus and MTL, typically reporting a decrease in hippocampal or parahippocampal activity during information encoding.[130–134] Moreover, several studies

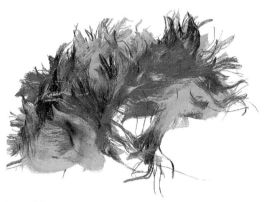

Fig. 3. Reconstruction of intracortically projecting fiber tracts from diffusion spectrum imaging of a healthy woman, 50 years of age, during a half-scheme acquisition of 256 gradient directions with an acquisition time of 30 minutes. Colors indicate the main direction of fiber tracts in left-right (*red*), superior-inferior (*blue*) and anterior-posterior (*green*) directions. Fiber tracts have been reconstructed using DSI-Studio software (developed by Fang-Cheng Yeh, Department of Biomedical Engineering, Carnegie Mellon University; www.dsi-studio.labsolver.org) with default parameters.

have reported a decreased activation in the MTL in patients with MCI.[135–137] A substantial body of fMRI research has focused on the "default network," that is, the interplay between a particular set of cortical regions and the hippocampal memory system,[138] whose activity is thought to decrease when assisting encoding (eg, during memory-intensive tasks) and to increase during information retrieval.[139] Accordingly, several investigators have reported dysfunctional modulation of encoding-related network activity in AD.[135,140–143] Also, resting-state fMRI (rsfMRI) is rapidly gaining ground as a technique able to reveal subtle changes in brain functional connectivity, and several rsfMRI studies have been able to demonstrate altered default-mode activity in AD patients[144–148] as well as in MCI, in which case it has been associated with a higher risk of converting to AD-related dementia.[149] A large (underexploited) potential of fMRI or rsfMRI in AD and MCI may be the longitudinal prediction of disease progression for devising novel treatment strategies. Although it is known that fMRI can detect drug-induced modulation of memory-related networks,[150] to date only a few studies have demonstrated altered activation after, for example, long-term treatment with cholinesterase inhibitors in MCI and AD,[151–154] and the potential of rsfMRI studies in elucidating acute and chronic drug-related alterations in function and connectivity has yet to be fully explored.[155]

Complexity-Based Indicators of Disease

In the search for novel, synthetic descriptors of brain structure and function able to extract additional information from data provided by existing MR protocols, the concept of complexity (either structural or functional) seems particularly promising. Physiologic systems manifest complex nonstationary and nonlinear behavior, and several studies have unveiled a general reduction of complexity with aging and disease in different physiologic systems.[156,157] Accordingly it has been shown that nonlinear analyses using concepts such as entropy, fractality, and predictability can offer significant diagnostic and prognostic information on several systemic and central nervous system disorders.[158–160] The brain cortex is statistically self-similar (fractal) down to the scale of 2.5 mm, which approximately coincides with cortical thickness.[161] Hence, the fractal dimension (FD) of cortical gray matter (as estimated based on T1-weighted MRI) can be seen as a multiscale descriptor of the overall size of the brain as well as the size of the folded cortex. FD has been found to be nonuniformly distributed between genders and across brain hemispheres[147] and is significantly reduced in aging patients,[162] those with multiple sclerosis,[163] and preterm infants with intrauterine growth restriction.[164] A few recent studies found a reduction of FD in early AD,[165,166] and multifractal analysis[167] unveiled age-related microstructural changes in the white matter in the frontal region, whose degree was associated with executive cognitive decline.[168] Significant differences in specific fractal descriptors of fMRI time series have been revealed in several cortical brain areas when comparing patients with early AD and controls,[169] and in a similar comparison higher regional fMRI signal entropy was associated with better cognitive performance.[170] In rsfMRI studies, a decreased mean level of functional connectivity as well as diminished fluctuations in the level of synchronization have been demonstrated in AD,[160] and the application of graphic theoretical analyses to the study of AD and other dementias has recently revealed the disruption of small-world network characteristics typical of healthy functional organization.[171]

Multimodal Data-Processing Strategies and Machine-Learning Techniques

The integration of the complementary information afforded by multimodal imaging protocols into a comprehensive analysis strategy is likely to aid in better discrimination and staging of AD,[172] and technical efforts are under way to devise optimized imaging protocols including state-of-the-art assessment of brain function, structure, micro-architecture, and quantitative parameters within a clinically feasible protocol.[173] Accordingly an increasing body of research has focused on methodological develop-ments that combine multimodal brain-imaging protocols in a multiparametric fashion[174–176] to formulate integrated hypotheses about structure-function links in both healthy and diseased brains. Although conventional statistical approaches allow articulate studies of statistical group differences as well as time-group interactions, their stand-alone use cannot allocate a single subject to a particular group on MR examination, hence limiting the overall diagnostic potential in a clinical setting. An extension of univariate logistic regression and discriminant analysis approaches for the construction of diagnostic models from region-driven or data-driven data is given by multivariate pattern classification techniques, including principal component anal-ysis and machine-learning algorithms such as support vector machines.[177–179] Such techniques have recently been identified as promising tools in neuroimaging data analysis,[180] especially because they are able to manage images from different modal-ities simultaneously and, importantly, to classify a single subject into a predefined group (eg, diseased or control group). Crucially, any type of data feature (eg, clinical, genetic, neuropsychological, and structural/functional neuroimaging data) can be integrated into the classification procedure, and the classification performance is not significantly degraded if same-modality data are collected in different centers and/or with different hardware.[180] In the context of atrophy quantification, machine-learning techniques make optimal use of the data by extracting and recognizing diagnosis-specific regional patterns of atrophy from preprocessed imaging data in an unsupervised manner, and can distinguish between AD patients, MCI subjects, and controls with high diagnostic accuracy. When trained to recognize spatial patterns of brain atrophy that best distinguish between AD patients and controls, pattern clas-sifiers can detect prodromal AD pathology in MCI subjects with accuracies of around 80%,[181] and may be used to assess an individual's risk for future cognitive decline.[182] Preliminary studies based on multimodal neuroimaging have also obtained promising results in discriminating AD and MCI patients.[183,184] Machine-learning algorithms are already now being developed for the software of scanner consoles as radiologic expert systems based on anatomic MRI data. In the future, these algorithms may be expanded to integrate diverse information from a multitude of image and biomarker modalities to improve the automated detection of prodromal AD stages based on high-dimensional pattern recognition.

SUMMARY

Hippocampus volumetry currently is the best-established imaging biomarker for AD. However, the effect of multicenter acquisition on measurements of hippocampus volume needs to be explicitly considered when it is applied in large clinical trials, for example by using mixed-effects models to take the clustering of data within centers into account.[185] The marker needs further validation in respect of the underlying neurobiological substrate and potential confounds such as vascular disease, inflammation, hydrocephalus, and alcoholism, and with regard to clinical outcomes such as cognition but also to demographic and socioeconomic outcomes such as mortality and institutionalization. The use of hippocampus volumetry for risk stratification of pre-dementia study samples will further increase with the availability of automated measurement approaches. An important step in this respect will be the development of a standard hippocampus tracing protocol that harmonizes the large range of presently available manual protocols.[44] In the near future, regionally differentiated automated methods will become available together with an appropriate statistical model, such as multivariate analysis of deformation fields, or techniques such as cortical-thickness measurements that yield a meaningful metrics for the detection of treatment effects. More advanced imaging protocols, including DTI, DSI, and functional MRI, are presently being used in monocenter and first multicenter studies. In the future these techniques will be relevant for the risk stratification in phase IIa type studies (small proof-of-concept trials). By contrast, the application of the broader established structural imaging biomarkers, such as hippocampus volume, for risk stratification and as surrogate end point is already today part of many clinical trial protocols. However, clinical care will also be affected by these new technologies. Radiologic expert centers already offer "dementia screening" for well-off middle-aged people who undergo an MRI scan with subsequent automated, typically VBM-based analysis, and determination of z-score deviation from a matched control cohort. Next-generation scanner software will likely include radiologic expert systems for automated segmentation, deformation-based morphometry, and multivariate analysis of anatomic MRI scans for the detection of a typical AD pattern. As these developments will start to change medical practice, first for selected subject groups that can afford this type of screening but later eventually also for other cohorts, clinicians must become aware of the potentials and limitations of these technologies. It is decidedly unclear to date how a middle-aged cognitively intact subject with a seemingly AD-positive MRI scan should be clinically advised. There is no evidence for individual risk prediction and even less for specific treatments. Thus, the development of preclinical diagnostic imaging poses not only technical but also ethical problems that must be critically discussed on the basis of profound knowledge.

From a neurobiological point of view, the main determinants of cognitive impairment in AD are the density of synapses and neurons in distributed cortical and subcortical networks.[186] MRI-based measures of regional gray matter volume and associated multivariate analysis techniques of regional interactions of gray matter densities provide insight into the onset and temporal dynamics of cortical atrophy as a close proxy for regional neuronal loss[187] and a basis of functional impairment in specific neuronal networks.[188] From the clinical point of view, clinicians must bear in mind that patients do not suffer from hippocampus atrophy or disconnection but from memory impairment, and that dementia screening in asymptomatic subjects should not be used outside of clinical studies.

REFERENCES

1. Braak H, Braak E. Staging of Alzheimer's disease-related neurofibrillary changes. Neurobiol Aging 1995;16(3):271–8 [discussion: 278–84].
2. Thal DR, Capetillo-Zarate E, Del Tredici K, et al. The development of amyloid beta protein deposits in the aged brain. Sci Aging Knowledge Environ 2006; 2006(6):re1.
3. Albert MS, DeKosky ST, Dickson D, et al. The diagnosis of mild cognitive impairment due to Alzheimer's disease: recommendations from the National Institute on Aging—Alzheimer's Association workgroups on diagnostic guidelines for Alzheimer's disease. Alzheimers Dement 2011;7(3):270–9.
4. Dubois B, Feldman HH, Jacova C, et al. Revising the definition of Alzheimer's disease: a new lexicon. Lancet Neurol 2010;9(11):1118–27.
5. Sperling RA, Aisen PS, Beckett LA, et al. Toward defining the preclinical stages of Alzheimer's disease: recommendations from the National Institute on Aging—Alzheimer's Association workgroups on diagnostic guidelines for Alzheimer's disease. Alzheimers Dement 2011;7(3):280–92.
6. McKhann G, Drachman D, Folstein M, et al. Clinical diagnosis of Alzheimer's disease: report of the NINCDS-ADRDA Work Group under the auspices of the Department of Health and Human Services Task Force on Alzheimer's disease. Neurology 1984;34:939–44.
7. McKhann GM, Albert MS, Grossman M, et al. Clinical and pathological diagnosis of frontotemporal dementia: report of the Work Group on Frontotemporal Dementia and Pick's Disease. Arch Neurol 2001;58(11):1803–9.
8. Golde TE. Alzheimer disease therapy: can the amyloid cascade be halted? J Clin Invest 2003;111(1):11–8.
9. Bobinski M, de Leon MJ, Wegiel J, et al. The histological validation of post mortem magnetic resonance imaging-determined hippocampal volume in Alzheimer's disease. Neuroscience 2000;95(3):721–5.
10. Giannakopoulos P, Kovari E, Gold G, et al. Pathological substrates of cognitive decline in Alzheimer's disease. Front Neurol Neurosci 2009;24:20–9.
11. Hampel H, Frank R, Broich K, et al. Biomarkers for Alzheimer's disease: academic, industry and regulatory perspectives. Nat Rev Drug Discov 2010; 9(7):560–74.
12. Giedd JN, Kozuch P, Kaysen D, et al. Reliability of cerebral measures in repeated examinations with magnetic resonance imaging. Psychiatry Res 1995;61(2):113–9.
13. Byrum CE, MacFall JR, Charles HC, et al. Accuracy and reproducibility of brain and tissue volumes using a magnetic resonance segmentation method. Psychiatry Res 1996;67(3):215–34.
14. Ewers M, Teipel SJ, Dietrich O, et al. Multicenter assessment of reliability of cranial MRI. Neurobiol Aging 2006;27(8):1051–9.
15. Zarow C, Vinters HV, Ellis WG, et al. Correlates of hippocampal neuron number in Alzheimer's disease and ischemic vascular dementia. Ann Neurol 2005;57(6):896–903.

16. Freeman SH, Kandel R, Cruz L, et al. Preservation of neuronal number despite age-related cortical brain atrophy in elderly subjects without Alzheimer disease. J Neuropathol Exp Neurol 2008;67(12):1205–12.

17. Scheltens P, Leys D, Barkhof F, et al. Atrophy of medial temporal lobes on MRI in "probable" Alzheimer's disease and normal ageing: diagnostic value and neuropsychological correlates. J Neurol Neurosurg Psychiatr 1992;55:967–72.

18. Wahlund LO, Julin P, Johansson SE, et al. Visual rating and volumetry of the medial temporal lobe on magnetic resonance imaging in dementia: a comparative study. J Neurol Neurosurg Psychiatr 2000;69(5):630–5.

19. Ridha BH, Barnes J, van de Pol LA, et al. Application of automated medial temporal lobe atrophy scale to Alzheimer disease. Arch Neurol 2007;64(6): 849–54.

20. Bresciani L, Rossi R, Testa C, et al. Visual assessment of medial temporal atrophy on MR films in Alzheimer's disease: comparison with volumetry. Aging Clin Exp Res 2005;17(1):8–13.

21. Seab JP, Jagust WJ, Wong ST, et al. Quantitative NMR measurements of hippocampal atrophy in Alzheimer's disease. Magn Reson Med 1988;8(2):200–8.

22. Killiany RJ, Moss MB, Albert MS, et al. Temporal lobe regions on magnetic resonance imaging identify patients with early Alzheimer's disease. Arch Neurol 1993;50(9):949–54.

23. Csernansky JG, Hamstra J, Wang L, et al. Correlations between antemortem hippocampal volume and postmortem neuropathology in AD subjects. Alzheimer Dis Assoc Disord 2004;18(4):190–5.

24. Lehericy S, Baulac M, Chiras J, et al. Amygdalohippocampal MR volume measurements in the early stages of Alzheimer's disease. AJNR Am J Neuroradiol 1994;15:927–37.

25. Teipel SJ, Pruessner JC, Faltraco F, et al. Comprehensive dissection of the medial temporal lobe in AD: measurement of hippocampus, amygdala, entorhinal, perirhinal and parahippocampal cortices using MRI. J Neurol 2006;253(6):794–800.

26. Rusinek H, de Leon MJ, George AE, et al. Alzheimer disease: measuring loss of cerebral gray matter with MR imaging. Radiology 1991;178(1):109–14.

27. Teipel SJ, Bayer W, Alexander GE, et al. Regional pattern of hippocampus and corpus callosum atrophy in Alzheimer's disease in relation to dementia severity: evidence for early neocortical degeneration. Neurobiol Aging 2003;24(1):85–94.

28. Petersen RC. Mild cognitive impairment as a diagnostic entity. J Intern Med 2004;256(3):183–94.

29. Guillozet AL, Weintraub S, Mash DC, et al. Neurofibrillary tangles, amyloid, and memory in aging and mild cognitive impairment. Arch Neurol 2003;60(5): 729–36.

30. Convit A, De Leon MJ, Tarshish C, et al. Specific hippocampal volume reductions in individuals at risk for Alzheimer's disease. Neurobiol Aging 1997; 18(2):131–8.

31. Convit A, de Asis J, de Leon MJ, et al. Atrophy of the medial occipitotemporal, inferior, and middle temporal gyri in non-demented elderly predict decline to Alzheimer's disease. Neurobiol Aging 2000;21(1):19–26.

32. Du AT, Schuff N, Amend D, et al. Magnetic resonance imaging of the entorhinal cortex and hippocampus in mild cognitive impairment and Alzheimer's disease. J Neurol Neurosurg Psychiatr 2001;71(4):441–7.

33. Jack CR Jr, Petersen RC, Xu YC, et al. Prediction of AD with MRI-based hippocampal volume in mild cognitive impairment. Neurology 1999;52(7): 1397–403.

34. Killiany RJ, Hyman BT, Gomez-Isla T, et al. MRI measures of entorhinal cortex vs hippocampus in preclinical AD. Neurology 2002;58(8):1188–96.

35. deToledo-Morrell L, Stoub TR, Bulgakova M, et al. MRI-derived entorhinal volume is a good predictor of conversion from MCI to AD. Neurobiol Aging 2004;25(9):1197–203.

36. Devanand DP, Pradhaban G, Liu X, et al. Hippocampal and entorhinal atrophy in mild cognitive impairment: prediction of Alzheimer disease. Neurology 2007; 68(11):828–36.

37. Krasuski JS, Alexander GE, Horwitz B, et al. Volumes of medial temporal lobe structures in patients with Alzheimer's disease and mild cognitive impairment (and in healthy controls). Biol Psychiatry 1998;43:60–8.

38. Pennanen C, Kivipelto M, Tuomainen S, et al. Hippocampus and entorhinal cortex in mild cognitive impairment and early AD. Neurobiol Aging 2004; 25(3):303–10.

39. Xu Y, Jack CR Jr, O'Brien PC, et al. Usefulness of MRI measures of entorhinal cortex versus hippocampus in AD. Neurology 2000;54(9):1760–7.

40. Risacher SL, Saykin AJ, West JD, et al. Baseline MRI predictors of conversion from MCI to probable AD in the ADNI cohort. Curr Alzheimer Res 2009;6(4): 347–61.

41. Kaye JA, Swihart T, Howieson D, et al. Volume loss of the hippocampus and temporal lobe in healthy elderly persons destined to develop dementia. Neurology 1997;48(5):1297–304.

42. den Heijer T, Geerlings MI, Hoebeek FE, et al. Use of hippocampal and amygdalar volumes on magnetic resonance imaging to predict dementia in cognitively intact elderly people. Arch Gen Psychiatry 2006;63(1):57–62.

43. Martin SB, Smith CD, Collins HR, et al. Evidence that volume of anterior medial temporal lobe is reduced in seniors destined for mild cognitive impairment. Neurobiol Aging 2010;31(7):1099–106.

44. Frisoni GB, Jack CR. Harmonization of magnetic resonance-based manual hippocampal segmentation: a mandatory step for wide clinical use. Alzheimers Dement 2011;7(2):171–4.

45. Chupin M, Gerardin E, Cuingnet R, et al. Fully automatic hippocampus segmentation and classification in Alzheimer's disease and mild cognitive impairment applied on data from ADNI. Hippocampus 2009;19(6):579–87.

46. Mueller SG, Weiner MW. Selective effect of age, Apo e4, and Alzheimer's disease on hippocampal subfields. Hippocampus 2009;19(6):558–64.

47. Hanseeuw BJ, Van Leemput K, Kavec M, et al. Mild cognitive impairment: differential atrophy in the hippocampal subfields. AJNR Am J Neuroradiol 2011;32(9): 1658–61.

48. Kerchner GA, Deutsch GK, Zeineh M, et al. Hippocampal CA1 apical neuropil atrophy and memory performance in Alzheimer's disease. Neuroimage 2012; 63(1):194–202.

49. Wang L, Beg F, Ratnanather T, et al. Large deformation diffeomorphism and momentum based hippocampal shape discrimination in dementia of the Alzheimer type. IEEE Trans Med Imaging 2007;26(4):462–70.

50. Gerardin E, Chetelat G, Chupin M, et al. Multidimensional classification of hippocampal shape features discriminates Alzheimer's disease and mild cognitive impairment from normal aging. Neuroimage 2009;47(4):1476–86.

51. Tondelli M, Wilcock GK, Nichelli P, et al. Structural MRI changes detectable up to ten years before clinical Alzheimer's disease. Neurobiol Aging 2012;33(4): 825.e25–36.

52. Ashburner J, Friston KJ. Voxel-based morphometry—the methods. Neuroimage 2000;11(6 Pt 1):805–21.
53. Fischl B, van der Kouwe A, Destrieux C, et al. Automatically parcellating the human cerebral cortex. Cereb Cortex 2004;14(1):11–22.
54. Klein A, Andersson J, Ardekani BA, et al. Evaluation of 14 nonlinear deformation algorithms applied to human brain MRI registration. Neuroimage 2009;46(3): 786–802.
55. Leung KK, Barnes J, Ridgway GR, et al. Automated cross-sectional and longitudinal hippocampal volume measurement in mild cognitive impairment and Alzheimer's disease. Neuroimage 2010;51(4):1345–59.
56. Colliot O, Chetelat G, Chupin M, et al. Discrimination between Alzheimer disease, mild cognitive impairment, and normal aging by using automated segmentation of the hippocampus. Radiology 2008;248(1):194–201.
57. Mak HK, Zhang Z, Yau KK, et al. Efficacy of voxel-based morphometry with DARTEL and standard registration as imaging biomarkers in Alzheimer's disease patients and cognitively normal older adults at 3.0 Tesla MR imaging. J Alzheimers Dis 2011;23(4):655–64.
58. Calvini P, Chincarini A, Gemme G, et al. Automatic analysis of medial temporal lobe atrophy from structural MRIs for the early assessment of Alzheimer disease. Med Phys 2009;36(8):3737–47.
59. Desikan RS, Cabral HJ, Hess CP, et al. Automated MRI measures identify individuals with mild cognitive impairment and Alzheimer's disease. Brain 2009; 132(Pt 8):2048–57.
60. Lerch JP, Pruessner J, Zijdenbos AP, et al. Automated cortical thickness measurements from MRI can accurately separate Alzheimer's patients from normal elderly controls. Neurobiol Aging 2008;29(1):23–30.
61. Querbes O, Aubry F, Pariente J, et al. Early diagnosis of Alzheimer's disease using cortical thickness: impact of cognitive reserve. Brain 2009;132(Pt 8):2036–47.
62. Bakkour A, Morris JC, Dickerson BC. The cortical signature of prodromal AD: regional thinning predicts mild AD dementia. Neurology 2009;72(12):1048–55.
63. Bookstein FL. "Voxel-based morphometry" should not be used with imperfectly registered images. Neuroimage 2001;14(6):1454–62.
64. Ashburner J, Friston KJ. Why voxel-based morphometry should be used. Neuroimage 2001;14(6):1238–43.
65. Whitwell JL, Josephs KA, Murray ME, et al. MRI correlates of neurofibrillary tangle pathology at autopsy: a voxel-based morphometry study. Neurology 2008;71(10):743–9.
66. Di Paola M, Macaluso E, Carlesimo GA, et al. Episodic memory impairment in patients with Alzheimer's disease is correlated with entorhinal cortex atrophy. A voxel-based morphometry study. J Neurol 2007;254(6):774–81.
67. Grossman M, McMillan C, Moore P, et al. What's in a name: voxel-based morphometric analyses of MRI and naming difficulty in Alzheimer's disease, frontotemporal dementia and corticobasal degeneration. Brain 2004;127(Pt 3):628–49.
68. Josephs KA, Whitwell JL, Duffy JR, et al. Progressive aphasia secondary to Alzheimer disease vs FTLD pathology. Neurology 2008;70(1):25–34.
69. Gee J, Ding L, Xie Z, et al. Alzheimer's disease and frontotemporal dementia exhibit distinct atrophy-behavior correlates: a computer-assisted imaging study. Acad Radiol 2003;10(12):1392–401.
70. Frisoni GB, Testa C, Zorzan A, et al. Detection of grey matter loss in mild Alzheimer's disease with voxel based morphometry. J Neurol Neurosurg Psychiatr 2002;73(6):657–64.

71. Karas GB, Burton EJ, Rombouts SA, et al. A comprehensive study of gray matter loss in patients with Alzheimer's disease using optimized voxel-based morphometry. Neuroimage 2003;18(4):895–907.
72. Whitwell JL, Przybelski SA, Weigand SD, et al. 3D maps from multiple MRI illustrate changing atrophy patterns as subjects progress from mild cognitive impairment to Alzheimer's disease. Brain 2007;130(Pt 7):1777–86.
73. Ries ML, Carlsson CM, Rowley HA, et al. Magnetic resonance imaging characterization of brain structure and function in mild cognitive impairment: a review. J Am Geriatr Soc 2008;56(5):920–34.
74. Chetelat G, Landeau B, Eustache F, et al. Using voxel-based morphometry to map the structural changes associated with rapid conversion in MCI: a longitudinal MRI study. Neuroimage 2005;27(4):934–46.
75. Risacher SL, Shen L, West JD, et al. Longitudinal MRI atrophy biomarkers: relationship to conversion in the ADNI cohort. Neurobiol Aging 2010;31(8):1401–18.
76. Hall AM, Moore RY, Lopez OL, et al. Basal forebrain atrophy is a presymptomatic marker for Alzheimer's disease. Alzheimers Dement 2008;4(4):271–9.
77. Driscoll I, Davatzikos C, An Y, et al. Longitudinal pattern of regional brain volume change differentiates normal aging from MCI. Neurology 2009;72(22):1906–13.
78. Csernansky JG, Wang L, Swank J, et al. Preclinical detection of Alzheimer's disease: hippocampal shape and volume predict dementia onset in the elderly. Neuroimage 2005;25(3):783–92.
79. Heckemann RA, Keihaninejad S, Aljabar P, et al. Automatic morphometry in Alzheimer's disease and mild cognitive impairment. Neuroimage 2011;56(4):2024–37.
80. Barnes J, Foster J, Boyes RG, et al. A comparison of methods for the automated calculation of volumes and atrophy rates in the hippocampus. Neuroimage 2008;40(4):1655–71.
81. Bartus RT, Dean RL, Pontecorvo MJ, et al. The cholinergic hypothesis: a historical overview, current perspective, and future directions. Ann N Y Acad Sci 1985;444:332–58.
82. Mesulam M. The cholinergic lesion of Alzheimer's disease: pivotal factor or side show? Learn Mem 2004;11(1):43–9.
83. Huckman MS. Where's the chicken? AJNR Am J Neuroradiol 1995;16(10):2008–9.
84. Hanyu H, Asano T, Sakurai H, et al. MR analysis of the substantia innominata in normal aging, Alzheimer disease, and other types of dementia. AJNR Am J Neuroradiol 2002;23(1):27–32.
85. Teipel SJ, Flatz WH, Heinsen H, et al. Measurement of basal forebrain atrophy in Alzheimer's disease using MRI. Brain 2005;128(Pt 11):2626–44.
86. Zaborszky L, Hoemke L, Mohlberg H, et al. Stereotaxic probabilistic maps of the magnocellular cell groups in human basal forebrain. Neuroimage 2008;42(3):1127–41.
87. Grothe M, Heinsen H, Teipel SJ. Atrophy of the cholinergic basal forebrain over the adult age range and in early stages of Alzheimer's disease. Biol Psychiatry 2012;71(9):805–13.
88. Teipel SJ, Meindl T, Grinberg L, et al. The cholinergic system in mild cognitive impairment and Alzheimer's disease: an in vivo MRI and DTI study. Hum Brain Mapp 2011;32(9):1349–62.
89. Basser PJ, Jones DK. Diffusion-tensor MRI: theory, experimental design and data analysis—a technical review. NMR Biomed 2002;15(7–8):456–67.

90. Bozzali M, Cherubini A. Diffusion tensor MRI to investigate dementias: a brief review. Magn Reson Imaging 2007;25(6):969–77.
91. Chua TC, Wen W, Slavin MJ, et al. Diffusion tensor imaging in mild cognitive impairment and Alzheimer's disease: a review. Curr Opin Neurol 2008;21(1): 83–92.
92. Hess CP. Update on diffusion tensor imaging in Alzheimer's disease. Magn Reson Imaging Clin N Am 2009;17(2):215–24.
93. Jones DK, Leemans A. Diffusion tensor imaging. Methods Mol Biol 2011;711: 127–44.
94. Giannelli M, Belmonte G, Toschi N, et al. Technical note: DTI measurements of fractional anisotropy and mean diffusivity at 1.5 T: comparison of two radiofrequency head coils with different functional designs and sensitivities. Med Phys 2011;38(6):3205–11.
95. Jones DK. Studying connections in the living human brain with diffusion MRI. Cortex 2008;44(8):936–52.
96. Medina D, DeToledo-Morrell L, Urresta F, et al. White matter changes in mild cognitive impairment and AD: a diffusion tensor imaging study. Neurobiol Aging 2006;27(5):663–72.
97. Liu Y, Spulber G, Lehtimaki KK, et al. Diffusion tensor imaging and tract-based spatial statistics in Alzheimer's disease and mild cognitive impairment. Neurobiol Aging 2011;32(9):1558–71.
98. O'Dwyer L, Lamberton F, Bokde AL, et al. Multiple indices of diffusion identifies white matter damage in mild cognitive impairment and Alzheimer's disease. PLoS One 2011;6(6):e21745.
99. Fjell AM, Amlien IK, Westlye LT, et al. Mini-mental state examination is sensitive to brain atrophy in Alzheimer's disease. Dement Geriatr Cogn Disord 2009; 28(3):252–8.
100. Heo JH, Lee ST, Kon C, et al. White matter hyperintensities and cognitive dysfunction in Alzheimer disease. J Geriatr Psychiatry Neurol 2009;22(3): 207–12.
101. Teipel SJ, Meindl T, Wagner M, et al. Longitudinal changes in fiber tract integrity in healthy aging and mild cognitive impairment: a DTI follow-up study. J Alzheimers Dis 2010;22(2):507–22.
102. Chua TC, Wen W, Chen X, et al. Diffusion tensor imaging of the posterior cingulate is a useful biomarker of mild cognitive impairment. Am J Geriatr Psychiatry 2009;17(7):602–13.
103. Takahashi S, Yonezawa H, Takahashi J, et al. Selective reduction of diffusion anisotropy in white matter of Alzheimer disease brains measured by 3.0 Tesla magnetic resonance imaging. Neurosci Lett 2002;332(1):45–8.
104. Zhang L, Dean D, Liu JZ, et al. Quantifying degeneration of white matter in normal aging using fractal dimension. Neurobiol Aging 2007;28(10):1543–55.
105. Zhuang L, Wen W, Zhu W, et al. White matter integrity in mild cognitive impairment: a tract-based spatial statistics study. Neuroimage 2010;53(1):16–25.
106. Douaud G, Jbabdi S, Behrens TE, et al. DTI measures in crossing-fibre areas: increased diffusion anisotropy reveals early white matter alteration in MCI and mild Alzheimer's disease. Neuroimage 2011;55(3):880–90.
107. Ennis DB, Kindlmann G. Orthogonal tensor invariants and the analysis of diffusion tensor magnetic resonance images. Magn Reson Med 2006;55(1):136–46.
108. Stricker NH, Schweinsburg BC, Delano-Wood L, et al. Decreased white matter integrity in late-myelinating fiber pathways in Alzheimer's disease supports retrogenesis. Neuroimage 2009;45(1):10–6.

109. Teipel SJ, Stahl R, Dietrich O, et al. Multivariate network analysis of fiber tract integrity in Alzheimer's disease. Neuroimage 2007;34(3):985–95.

110. Sexton CE, Kalu UG, Filippini N, et al. A meta-analysis of diffusion tensor imaging in mild cognitive impairment and Alzheimer's disease. Neurobiol Aging 2011;32(12):2322.e5–e18.

111. Teipel SJ, Wegrzyn M, Meindl T, et al. Anatomical MRI and DTI in the diagnosis of Alzheimer's disease: a European multicenter Study. J Alzheimers Dis 2012; 31(0):S33–47.

112. Alexander AL, Hasan KM, Lazar M, et al. Analysis of partial volume effects in diffusion-tensor MRI. Magn Reson Med 2001;45(5):770–80.

113. Wedeen VJ, Wang RP, Schmahmann JD, et al. Diffusion spectrum magnetic resonance imaging (DSI) tractography of crossing fibers. Neuroimage 2008; 41(4):1267–77.

114. Fieremans E, Jensen JH, Helpern JA. White matter characterization with diffusional kurtosis imaging. Neuroimage 2011;58(1):177–88.

115. Hui ES, Cheung MM, Qi L, et al. Advanced MR diffusion characterization of neural tissue using directional diffusion kurtosis analysis. Conf Proc IEEE Eng Med Biol Soc 2008;2008:3941–4.

116. Jensen JH, Helpern JA. Progress in diffusion-weighted imaging: concepts, techniques and applications to the central nervous system. NMR Biomed 2010;23(7):659–60.

117. Alexander DC. Multiple-fiber reconstruction algorithms for diffusion MRI. Ann N Y Acad Sci 2005;1064:113–33.

118. Assaf Y, Blumenfeld-Katzir T, Yovel Y, et al. AxCaliber: a method for measuring axon diameter distribution from diffusion MRI. Magn Reson Med 2008;59(6): 1347–54.

119. Assaf Y, Basser PJ. Composite hindered and restricted model of diffusion (CHARMED) MR imaging of the human brain. Neuroimage 2005;27(1):48–58.

120. Alexander DC, Hubbard PL, Hall MG, et al. Orientationally invariant indices of axon diameter and density from diffusion MRI. Neuroimage 2010;52(4): 1374–89.

121. De Santis S, Gabrielli A, Bozzali M, et al. Anisotropic anomalous diffusion assessed in the human brain by scalar invariant indices. Magn Reson Med 2011;65(4):1043–52.

122. De Santis S, Gabrielli A, Palombo M, et al. Non-Gaussian diffusion imaging: a brief practical review. Magn Reson Imaging 2011;29(10):1410–6.

123. Mintun MA, Larossa GN, Sheline YI, et al. [^{11}C]PIB in a nondemented population: potential antecedent marker of Alzheimer disease. Neurology 2006;67(3): 446–52.

124. Iraji A, Davoodi-Bojd E, Soltanian-Zadeh H, et al. Diffusion kurtosis imaging discriminates patients with white matter lesions from healthy subjects. Conf Proc IEEE Eng Med Biol Soc 2011;2011:2796–9.

125. Falangola MF, Jensen JH, Babb JS, et al. Age-related non-Gaussian diffusion patterns in the prefrontal brain. J Magn Reson Imaging 2008;28(6):1345–50.

126. Wang JJ, Lin WY, Lu CS, et al. Parkinson disease: diagnostic utility of diffusion kurtosis imaging. Radiology 2011;261(1):210–7.

127. Bookheimer SY, Strojwas MH, Cohen MS, et al. Patterns of brain activation in people at risk for Alzheimer's disease. N Engl J Med 2000;343(7):450–6.

128. Borghesani PR, Johnson LC, Shelton AL, et al. Altered medial temporal lobe responses during visuospatial encoding in healthy APOE*4 carriers. Neurobiol Aging 2008;29(7):981–91.

129. Filippini N, MacIntosh BJ, Hough MG, et al. Distinct patterns of brain activity in young carriers of the APOE-epsilon4 allele. Proc Natl Acad Sci U S A 2009; 106(17):7209–14.

130. Golby A, Silverberg G, Race E, et al. Memory encoding in Alzheimer's disease: an fMRI study of explicit and implicit memory. Brain 2005;128(Pt 4):773–87.

131. Gron G, Bittner D, Schmitz B, et al. Hippocampal activations during repetitive learning and recall of geometric patterns. Learn Mem 2001;8(6):336–45.

132. Hamalainen A, Pihlajamaki M, Tanila H, et al. Increased fMRI responses during encoding in mild cognitive impairment. Neurobiol Aging 2007;28(12):1889–903.

133. Sperling R. Functional MRI studies of associative encoding in normal aging, mild cognitive impairment, and Alzheimer's disease. Ann N Y Acad Sci 2007; 1097:146–55.

134. Sperling RA, Dickerson BC, Pihlajamaki M, et al. Functional alterations in memory networks in early Alzheimer's disease. Neuromolecular Med 2010; 12(1):27–43.

135. Celone KA, Calhoun VD, Dickerson BC, et al. Alterations in memory networks in mild cognitive impairment and Alzheimer's disease: an independent component analysis. J Neurosci 2006;26(40):10222–31.

136. Johnson SC, Schmitz TW, Moritz CH, et al. Activation of brain regions vulnerable to Alzheimer's disease: the effect of mild cognitive impairment. Neurobiol Aging 2006;27(11):1604–12.

137. Petrella JR, Wang L, Krishnan S, et al. Cortical deactivation in mild cognitive impairment: high-field-strength functional MR imaging. Radiology 2007;245(1): 224–35.

138. Satterthwaite TD, Green L, Myerson J, et al. Dissociable but inter-related systems of cognitive control and reward during decision making: evidence from pupillometry and event-related fMRI. Neuroimage 2007;37(3):1017–31.

139. Vannini P, Hedden T, Becker JA, et al. Age and amyloid-related alterations in default network habituation to stimulus repetition. Neurobiol Aging 2012;33(7): 1237–52.

140. Fleisher AS, Sherzai A, Taylor C, et al. Resting-state BOLD networks versus task-associated functional MRI for distinguishing Alzheimer's disease risk groups. Neuroimage 2009;47(4):1678–90.

141. Pihlajamaki M, O'Keefe K, O'Brien J, et al. Failure of repetition suppression and memory encoding in aging and Alzheimer's disease. Brain Imaging Behav 2011; 5(1):36–44.

142. Pihlajamaki M, O'Keefe K, Bertram L, et al. Evidence of altered posteromedial cortical FMRI activity in subjects at risk for Alzheimer disease. Alzheimer Dis Assoc Disord 2010;24(1):28–36.

143. Pihlajamaki M, DePeau KM, Blacker D, et al. Impaired medial temporal repetition suppression is related to failure of parietal deactivation in Alzheimer disease. Am J Geriatr Psychiatry 2008;16(4):283–92.

144. Greicius MD, Srivastava G, Reiss AL, et al. Default-mode network activity distinguishes Alzheimer's disease from healthy aging: evidence from functional MRI. Proc Natl Acad Sci U S A 2004;101(13):4637–42.

145. Greicius MD, Supekar K, Menon V, et al. Resting-state functional connectivity reflects structural connectivity in the default mode network. Cereb Cortex 2009;19(1):72–8.

146. Sorg C, Riedl V, Muhlau M, et al. Selective changes of resting-state networks in individuals at risk for Alzheimer's disease. Proc Natl Acad Sci U S A 2007; 104(47):18760–5.

147. Wang K, Liang M, Wang L, et al. Altered functional connectivity in early Alzheimer's disease: a resting-state fMRI study. Hum Brain Mapp 2007;28(10): 967–78.
148. Wermke M, Sorg C, Wohlschlager AM, et al. A new integrative model of cerebral activation, deactivation and default mode function in Alzheimer's disease. Eur J Nucl Med Mol Imaging 2008;35(Suppl 1):S12–24.
149. Petrella JR, Sheldon FC, Prince SE, et al. Default mode network connectivity in stable vs progressive mild cognitive impairment. Neurology 2011;76(6): 511–7.
150. Kukolja J, Thiel CM, Fink GR. Cholinergic stimulation enhances neural activity associated with encoding but reduces neural activity associated with retrieval in humans. J Neurosci 2009;29(25):8119–28.
151. Goekoop R, Scheltens P, Barkhof F, et al. Cholinergic challenge in Alzheimer patients and mild cognitive impairment differentially affects hippocampal activation—a pharmacological fMRI study. Brain 2006;129(Pt 1):141–57.
152. Rombouts SA, Barkhof F, Van Meel CS, et al. Alterations in brain activation during cholinergic enhancement with rivastigmine in Alzheimer's disease. J Neurol Neurosurg Psychiatr 2002;73(6):665–71.
153. Saykin AJ, Wishart HA, Rabin LA, et al. Cholinergic enhancement of frontal lobe activity in mild cognitive impairment. Brain 2004;127(Pt 7):1574–83.
154. Shanks MF, McGeown WJ, Forbes-McKay KE, et al. Regional brain activity after prolonged cholinergic enhancement in early Alzheimer's disease. Magn Reson Imaging 2007;25(6):848–59.
155. Sperling R. Potential of functional MRI as a biomarker in early Alzheimer's disease. Neurobiol Aging 2011;32(Suppl 1):37–43.
156. Goldberger AL, Amaral LA, Hausdorff JM, et al. Fractal dynamics in physiology: alterations with disease and aging. Proc Natl Acad Sci U S A 2002;99(Suppl 1): 2466–72.
157. Goldberger AL, Peng CK, Lipsitz LA. What is physiologic complexity and how does it change with aging and disease? Neurobiol Aging 2002;23(1):23–6.
158. Andrzejak RG, Widman G, Lehnertz K, et al. The epileptic process as nonlinear deterministic dynamics in a stochastic environment: an evaluation on mesial temporal lobe epilepsy. Epilepsy Res 2001;44(2–3):129–40.
159. Osowski S, Swiderski B, Cichocki A, et al. Epileptic seizure characterization by Lyapunov exponent of EEG signal. Comput Methods Programs Biomed 2007; 26(5):1276–87.
160. Stam CJ, Montez T, Jones BF, et al. Disturbed fluctuations of resting state EEG synchronization in Alzheimer's disease. Clin Neurophysiol 2005;116(3):708–15.
161. Kiselev VG, Hahn KR, Auer DP. Is the brain cortex a fractal? Neuroimage 2003; 20(3):1765–74.
162. Zhang L, Liu JZ, Dean D, et al. A three-dimensional fractal analysis method for quantifying white matter structure in human brain. J Neurosci Methods 2006; 150(2):242–53.
163. Esteban FJ, Sepulcre J, de Mendizabal NV, et al. Fractal dimension and white matter changes in multiple sclerosis. Neuroimage 2007;36(3):543–9.
164. Esteban FJ, Padilla N, Sanz-Cortes M, et al. Fractal-dimension analysis detects cerebral changes in preterm infants with and without intrauterine growth restriction. Neuroimage 2010;53(4):1225–32.
165. King RD, George AT, Jeon T, et al. Characterization of atrophic changes in the cerebral cortex using fractal dimensional analysis. Brain Imaging Behav 2009; 3(2):154–66.

166. King RD, Brown B, Hwang M, et al. Fractal dimension analysis of the cortical ribbon in mild Alzheimer's disease. Neuroimage 2010;53(2):471–9.

167. Takahashi T, Murata T, Narita K, et al. Multifractal analysis of deep white matter microstructural changes on MRI in relation to early-stage atherosclerosis. Neuroimage 2006;32(3):1158–66.

168. Takahashi T, Murata T, Omori M, et al. Quantitative evaluation of age-related white matter microstructural changes on MRI by multifractal analysis. J Neurol Sci 2004;225(1–2):33–7.

169. Maxim V, Sendur L, Fadili J, et al. Fractional Gaussian noise, functional MRI and Alzheimer's disease. Neuroimage 2005;25(1):141–58.

170. Sokunbi MO, Staff RT, Waiter GD, et al. Inter-individual differences in fMRI entropy measurements in old age. IEEE Trans Biomed Eng 2011;58(11):3206–14.

171. Pievani M, de Haan W, Wu T, et al. Functional network disruption in the degenerative dementias. Lancet Neurol 2011;10(9):829–43.

172. Ewers M, Frisoni GB, Teipel SJ, et al. Staging Alzheimer's disease progression with multimodality neuroimaging. Prog Neurobiol 2011;95(4):535–46.

173. Landman BA, Huang AJ, Gifford A, et al. Multi-parametric neuroimaging reproducibility: a 3-T resource study. Neuroimage 2011;54(4):2854–66.

174. Casanova R, Srikanth R, Baer A, et al. Biological parametric mapping: a statistical toolbox for multimodality brain image analysis. Neuroimage 2007;34(1):137–43.

175. Oakes TR, Fox AS, Johnstone T, et al. Integrating VBM into the General Linear Model with voxelwise anatomical covariates. Neuroimage 2007;34(2):500–8.

176. Yang X, Beason-Held L, Resnick SM, et al. Biological parametric mapping with robust and non-parametric statistics. Neuroimage 2011;57(2):423–30.

177. Teipel SJ, Born C, Ewers M, et al. Multivariate deformation-based analysis of brain atrophy to predict Alzheimer's disease in mild cognitive impairment. Neuroimage 2007;38(1):13–24.

178. Plant C, Teipel SJ, Oswald A, et al. Automated detection of brain atrophy patterns based on MRI for the prediction of Alzheimer's disease. Neuroimage 2010;50(1):162–74.

179. Davatzikos C, Fan Y, Wu X, et al. Detection of prodromal Alzheimer's disease via pattern classification of MRI. Neurobiol Aging 2008;29(4):514–23.

180. Orru G, Pettersson-Yeo W, Marquand AF, et al. Using support vector machine to identify imaging biomarkers of neurological and psychiatric disease: a critical review. Neurosci Biobehav Rev 2012;36(4):1140–52.

181. Misra C, Fan Y, Davatzikos C. Baseline and longitudinal patterns of brain atrophy in MCI patients, and their use in prediction of short-term conversion to AD: results from ADNI. Neuroimage 2009;44(4):1415–22.

182. Davatzikos C, Xu F, An Y, et al. Longitudinal progression of Alzheimer's-like patterns of atrophy in normal older adults: the SPARE-AD index. Brain 2009;132(Pt 8):2026–35.

183. Zhang D, Shen D. Alzheimer's disease neuroimaging I. Multi-modal multi-task learning for joint prediction of multiple regression and classification variables in Alzheimer's disease. Neuroimage 2012;59(2):895–907.

184. Zhang D, Shen D. Alzheimer's disease neuroimaging I. Predicting future clinical changes of MCI patients using longitudinal and multimodal biomarkers. PLoS One 2012;7(3):e33182.

185. Teipel SJ, Ewers M, Wolf S, et al. Multicentre variability of MRI-based medial temporal lobe volumetry in Alzheimer's disease. Psychiatry Res 2011;182(3):244–50.

186. Giannakopoulos P, Herrmann FR, Bussiere T, et al. Tangle and neuron numbers, but not amyloid load, predict cognitive status in Alzheimer's disease. Neurology 2003;60(9):1495–500.
187. Smith AD. Commentary: imaging the progression of Alzheimer pathology through the brain. Proc Natl Acad Sci U S A 2002;99(7):4135–7.
188. Teipel SJ, Bokde AL, Born C, et al. The morphological substrate of face matching in healthy aging and mild cognitive impairment: a combined MRI-fMRI study. Brain 2007;130(Pt 7):1745–58.
189. Jack CR Jr, Petersen RC, Xu YC, et al. Medial temporal atrophy on MRI in normal aging and very mild Alzheimer's disease. Neurology 1997;49:786–94.
190. Wang PN, Lirng JF, Lin KN, et al. Prediction of Alzheimer's disease in mild cognitive impairment: a prospective study in Taiwan. Neurobiol Aging 2006;27(12):1797–806.
191. Barnes J, Bartlett JW, van de Pol LA, et al. A meta-analysis of hippocampal atrophy rates in Alzheimer's disease. Neurobiol Aging 2009;30(11):1711–23.
192. Raz N, Rodrigue KM, Head D, et al. Differential aging of the medial temporal lobe: a study of a five-year change. Neurology 2004;62(3):433–8.
193. Rusinek H, De Santi S, Frid D, et al. Regional brain atrophy rate predicts future cognitive decline: 6-year longitudinal MR imaging study of normal aging. Radiology 2003;229(3):691–6.
194. Kovacevic S, Rafii MS, Brewer JB. High-throughput, fully automated volumetry for prediction of MMSE and CDR decline in mild cognitive impairment. Alzheimer Dis Assoc Disord 2009;23(2):139–45.
195. Antharam V, Collingwood JF, Bullivant JP, et al. High field magnetic resonance microscopy of the human hippocampus in Alzheimer's disease: quantitative imaging and correlation with iron. Neuroimage 2012;59(2):1249–60.
196. Pluta J, Yushkevich P, Das S, et al. In vivo analysis of hippocampal subfield atrophy in mild cognitive impairment via semi-automatic segmentation of T2-weighted MRI. J Alzheimers Dis 2012;31(1):85–99.
197. Stoub TR, Bulgakova M, Leurgans S, et al. MRI predictors of risk of incident Alzheimer disease: a longitudinal study. Neurology 2005;64(9):1520–4.
198. Devanand DP, Liu X, Tabert MH, et al. Combining early markers strongly predicts conversion from mild cognitive impairment to Alzheimer's disease. Biol Psychiatry 2008;64(10):871–9.
199. Ezekiel F, Chao L, Kornak J, et al. Comparisons between global and focal brain atrophy rates in normal aging and Alzheimer disease: boundary Shift Integral versus tracing of the entorhinal cortex and hippocampus. Alzheimer Dis Assoc Disord 2004;18(4):196–201.
200. Fox NC, Cousens S, Scahill R, et al. Using serial registered brain magnetic resonance imaging to measure disease progression in Alzheimer disease: power calculations and estimates of sample size to detect treatment effects. Arch Neurol 2000;57(3):339–44.
201. Schott JM, Price SL, Frost C, et al. Measuring atrophy in Alzheimer disease: a serial MRI study over 6 and 12 months. Neurology 2005;65(1):119–24.
202. Smith CD, Chebrolu H, Wekstein DR, et al. Brain structural alterations before mild cognitive impairment. Neurology 2007;68(16):1268–73.
203. Thompson PM, Hayashi KM, Dutton RA, et al. Tracking Alzheimer's disease. Ann N Y Acad Sci 2007;1097:183–214.
204. Lerch JP, Pruessner JC, Zijdenbos A, et al. Focal decline of cortical thickness in Alzheimer's disease identified by computational neuroanatomy. Cereb Cortex 2005;15(7):995–1001.

Cognitive Approaches to Early Alzheimer's Disease Diagnosis

John Harrison, CSci, CPsychol, PhD

KEYWORDS

- Dementia screening • Mild cognitive impairment • Episodic memory
- Cognitive assessment • Alzheimer disease

KEY POINTS

- Many of the available tests usefully distinguish between normal healthy individuals and confirmed cases of Alzheimer disease (AD), but their capacity to distinguish cases of AD from other forms of dementia is typically poor.
- Furthermore, there is a need to identify individuals early in the disease process.
- Traditional 'paper-and pencil' measures tend to lack reliability and stability and are therefore unlikely to be fit for purpose as serial measures of cognitive change.

INTRODUCTION

The challenge for any reviewer of cognitive screening is to make a useful contribution beyond the excellent previously published reviews.[1] The cognitive domains known to be impaired in early Alzheimer disease (AD) have been well covered by investigators such as Rentz and Weintraub.[2] A summary of their observations and findings is included in **Table 1**. For many years, the field was missing a thorough review of the paradigms and technologies available for cognitive screening. However, this was in large part remedied by a thorough and well-documented review published by Ashford.[3] This seminal review focused on the use and content of the mini-mental state examination (MMSE) but also:

- Consideration of the pros and cons of dementia screening
- Regulatory guidance with respect to criteria for selecting measures ("simple, safe, precise and validated")
- The inadequacies of many available screening instruments
- The application of modern test theory to cognition screening
- A decision model for deciding whether to screen

Ashford makes the case for better detection of "memory dysfunction, MCI [mild cognitive impairment] and AD" (p.422) and argues for annual screening at age 75 years

Department of Medicine, Imperial College, London & Metis Cognition Ltd, Park House, Kilmington Common, Wiltshire BA12 6QY, UK
E-mail address: john@metiscog.com

Med Clin N Am 97 (2013) 425–438
http://dx.doi.org/10.1016/j.mcna.2012.12.014
0025-7125/13/$ – see front matter © 2013 Elsevier Inc. All rights reserved.

Table 1	
Rentz and Weintraub review of cognitive changes in early AD by domain	
Cognitive Domain	**Reference**
Episodic memory	26–31
Implicit memory	32,33
Language	34
Attention	35
Working memory	36,37
Visuospatial function	38
Executive function	37–40

Data from Rentz D, Weintraub S. Neuropsychological detection of early Alzheimer's disease. Scinto L, Daffner K, editors. Early diagnosis of Alzheimer's disease. 2000. p. 169–89.

and "as early as 60 years of age depending on risk factors". In his consideration of future perspectives, Ashford suggests that "Computerized testing and the Internet are extremely fertile opportunities". Recent experience shows Ashford's view to have been prophetic, and since the publication of his review, there has been a marked increase in the number of computerized and paper-and-pencil screening measures being offered. Ashford took the opportunity to reproduce as an appendix to his article the Brief Alzheimer Screen.[4]

Three key elements of any new review of cognitive approaches to early AD diagnosis should be to:

1. Identify the cognitive domains known to be compromised early in the disease process
2. Review the efficiency of the traditional measures proposed for use
3. Examine the claims made for computerized testing

Much of this information has previously been provided, and in the case of issues 2 and 3, by Ashford[3] and Snyder and colleagues[5] in particular. However, there are still some opportunity to contribute further. For example, some of the test owners and investigators approached by the PAD2020 group opted not to contribute to their review process. In many cases, it seems likely that this was because no specific claims were being made for the usefulness of instruments identified in the literature review for cognitive screening. Other owners and investigators may have chosen not to participate for several reasons, including the time and effort required to complete the PAD2020 documentation. This review includes an evaluation of some of the technologies for which data were not returned to the PAD2020 group.

A further issue for consideration is the value of single, cross-sectional evaluations of cognitive function versus repeated, serial assessment. Most methods of screening for early AD have sought to determine whether there is evidence of impairment in an individual with respect to expected performance based on normative data. However, such an approach captures only individuals who have reached a critical level of impairment. Psychologists working in clinical practice have typically selected less than 1.96 standard deviations (SDs) below mean performance as the threshold for deciding that any single individual's test score is prima facie evidence of impairment. This strategy is an extension of the logic for selecting a 1-tailed α level of 0.05 for testing significance, because −1.96 SDs equates to the point at which 5% of the population are expected to perform. Often, the cutoff is set more liberally when screening for drug trials, typically at a level of −1.5 SDs, but sometimes at the −1.00 SD level. Whatever the level selected, some proportion of the selected individuals perform at their true level of performance, which although low (ie, less than the cutoff score) does not imply the presence of disease, but is instead simply an indication of their usual level of performance. Thus studies recruit false-positive rates according to the cutoff used (**Table 2**).

Much of the current effort in developing pharmaceutical interventions for AD focuses on those in the prodromal stages of the disease. Here a single cutoff value at or less than −1.5 SDs runs the risk of missing those of most interest. As an example of this issue, take the hypothetical example of 2 individuals of interest. One is initially very cognitively able, and at first assessment performs at a level +3 SD higher than mean performance. However, 1 year later his performance has fallen to a level +1 SD more than the mean. In contrast, take the example of an individual whose true level of performance is at a level −2 SD less than the mean (ie, who naturally performs at a level lower than the usual cutoff threshold for determining impaired performance). A consideration of these 2 examples suggests that using a cutoff of −1.5 SD results in the inclusion of an individual without the disease of interest, whereas the individual whose cognition has declined by 2 SD is not included. Later in this article, the suitability of current screening tools for repeated assessment is considered. In advance of tackling cognition measurement, it seems prudent to begin with an account of the components of human cognition and some consideration of those are likely to be impaired in early AD.

THE ATOMS OF COGNITION

Much of our current conception of cognition is based on folk psychology. Thus, some of our core conceptual ideas are based on everyday terms such as memory, attention, language, and so forth. Late-nineteenth-century neuropsychologists showed that many of these domains are dissociable. Dissociable means that different individuals can show different patterns of cognitive impairment, often, but not reliably, by lesion location. For example, lesions to the hippocampus, as occurred in patient HM, can lead to difficulties with new memory formation.[6] Modern functional imaging has endorsed much of our understanding by showing activation in the same lesion areas in normal individuals who have been induced to use specific cognitive domains by experimental tasks. Contemporary neuropsychology, augmented by findings from experimental cognitive psychology, has furthered understanding of human cognition and it has been possible to some degree to refine ideas about specific domains of cognition. Accounts of the various atoms vary slightly, but for the most part have a clear family resemblance and are largely agreed on the cognitive atoms discussed in the following section.

Memory

The core of memory is that it reflects our capacity to encode, store, and retrieve information. The contribution of experimental cognitive psychology has been to show that memory can helpfully be further divided to aid our understanding. A full consideration is

Table 2
Proportion of the normal population captured by various commonly used cutoff points

Cutoff Used (SDs)	Proportion of Normal Population Captured (%)
−1.00	15.87
−1.5	11
−1.96	5

beyond the remit of this article, but one helpful distinction is the dissociation between episodic memory and semantic memory. Episodic memory relates to memory for events that have been experienced, autobiographical memories of times, places and information about who was present, what was done, and so forth. Semantic memory is composed of memory for concepts, factual information, and general knowledge. A further important component of memory is working memory. Working memory is understood to be a limited capacity online memory system in which concepts are literally brought to mind to assist problem solving. All memory systems decline as a function of disease progression in patients with AD. However, at least in the earliest stages, semantic memory is relatively preserved, although both episodic and working memory often show clear evidence of decline early in the disease process. Many of the screening tests used to assess patients focus on episodic memory, often using either word or paragraph learning tests, examples of which are shown in **Table 3**.

Praxis

This aspect of cognition concerns the individual's capacity to carry out movements. Conceptually, it is often further divided into several forms. As an example, ideational praxis requires the individual to successfully execute a motor program, such as to take a piece of paper in the right hand, fold it in half, and place it on the floor. Constructional praxis requires the participant to copy figures, such as circles, intersecting pentagons, three-dimensional cubes, and so forth. Praxis is also typically relatively well preserved in the early stages of AD, although patients in the moderate and severe stages of the disease (ie, with an MMSE score of <20) commonly show deficits.

Language

Several specific language deficits have been identified, including dissociations between the capacity to produce language and the ability to understand language. The language domain of cognition includes tests requiring individuals to name items according to rules (eg, words beginning with a certain letter or from a specific category, eg, animals), so-called phonologic fluency and semantic fluency tasks. When evaluating language, assessments of word finding difficulty and confrontation naming are also included. In confrontation naming, objects, or pictures of objects, are presented and individuals are challenged to name them.

Attention

A good working definition of attention is that it is the ability to focus on a specific aspect of our environment. The process is effortful, as is implicit in the expression "to pay attention", and is a limited resource. Like the cognitive domains discussed earlier, further helpful subdivisions can be made. For example, selective attention refers to the capacity to pay attention to a specific source of information. This function is often measured using tasks in which the individual must be vigilant in attending to a location

Table 3	
Commonly used episodic verbal memory measures	
Test Name	**Reference**
Free and Cued Selective Reminding Test	41
Wechsler Memory Scale Verbal Paired Associates Test	15
Wechsler Memory Scale Logical Memory Test	15
Hopkins Verbal Learning Test	42
Rey Auditory Verbal Learning Test	43

to which a stimulus is delivered. Common paradigms for assessing attention are so-called reaction time paradigms. In simple reaction time tasks, a predictable stimulus is delivered to a known location and the individual is asked to respond as quickly as possible on detecting the stimulus. Thus, by focusing and sustaining attention at the location, the individual can respond more quickly when the stimulus appears. Divided attention tasks require the individual to attend successfully to two or more sources of information and to switch attentional resources as the task requires.

Executive Function

Another cognitive domain is executive function. Executive function has proved to be a tricky area of cognition to define and there are myriad definitions. However, it is generally acknowledged that executive function is an umbrella terms that relates to the following cognitive skills and capacities:

- The ability to develop a strategy for problem solving
- Planning ahead
- Shifting between rules and concepts when engaged in problem solving
- Dealing with novelty
- The ability to inhibit specific behaviors or responses

Clarification of these subareas of executive function is often best achieved by providing examples of the kinds of paradigms we use to assess these skills. For example, a classic test of strategy and planning ahead is the tower of Hanoi puzzle, which features 3 pegs and a tower of 8 disks. The task requires that the individual transfers the 8 disks, which are of increasing size, to 1 of the other pegs in as few moves as possible. Disks can be moved only 1 at a time, and it is not allowed to place a larger disk onto a smaller one (**Fig. 1**). Successful completion requires the individual to develop a strategy and plan ahead to ensure completion in the minimum number of moves. A variety of tasks are used to evaluate set-shifting, and perhaps the simplest example is part B of the trail-making test. Here, individuals are required to connect a total of 25 circles on a piece of paper by drawing a continuous line. In part A of the test, the circles are numbered and must be connected in ascending sequence. However, in part B the circles can contain either numbers or letters and the task must be completed by connecting the circle labeled 1 to the circle labeled A, then 2 to B, 3 to C, and so forth. Thus, to successfully complete part B, it is necessary to alternate between letters and numbers, and to keep track of the last number and letter reached.

Most measures of cognitive screening in early AD feature the domains described earlier and some of the example tasks. In a later section, these cognitive domains are linked to standard AD screening measures. Before considering the various options for screening with cognition tests, it is helpful to consider the scope and purpose of

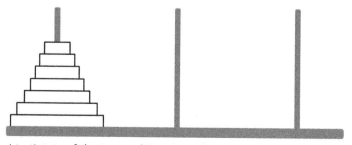

Fig. 1. The 'start' state of the tower of Hanoi problem.

cognitive screening. Poor performance on screening is used to after measures indi-cates cognitive impairment, although an important limitation is that these measures are typically mute regarding the cause of poor performance. As discussed earlier, in some instances, performance at or below the adopted impairment threshold can reflect the individual's true level of performance, although no pathologic process is at work. This is a major limitation of any screening program that relies on a single, cross-sectional analysis of performance, a topic returned to later. Cognition screening is also mute with respect to the specific disease process that has caused a change in cognitive status. For example, successful completion of episodic memory tests is believed to depend on the functional integrity of medial-temporal lobe structures, and especially the hippocampus. Changed or impaired performance on tests of episodic memory can be caused by damage to these anatomic structures. However, this damage could be caused by stroke, traumatic injury, infection, and so forth. Given this limitation, it seems unlikely that cognition measures will ever be diagnostic of any single pathologic process. Further, the current levels of sensitivity and specificity (typi-cally in the region of 90% for both metrics) seem unlikely to be significantly improved on. Increases in sensitivity can be achieved, but only at the cost of progressively decreasing levels of specificity (**Fig. 2** gives an example of the sensitivity and specificity of several commonly used cognition screening measures). Given these limitations, it is helpful to consider how and when cognition screening could be of assistance, a topic addressed in the following section.

WHAT NEED HAS TO BE MET?

Interest has been focused on the detection of cases of AD dissociated from individuals without the disease. In this context, traditional paper-and-pencil testing has usually

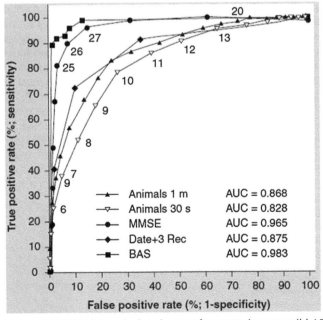

Fig. 2. Comparison of CERAD data calculated scores for control versus mild AD. (*Data from* Ashford JW. Screening for memory disorder, dementia, and Alzheimer's disease. Aging Health 2008;4(4):399–432.)

been adequate as a method of detecting cases of AD. However, recently, the requirement for detection has extended to interest in cases of prodromal AD. This stage of the disease has been extensively investigated in the past decade and the prodromal stage has acquired several epithets (see Ref.[7] for a helpful review), although most commentators seem to have settled on the term mild cognitive impairment (MCI). Studies of individuals with MCI that have compared performance with patients with confirmed AD and healthy controls (eg, Ref.[8]) have typically identified 3 distinct populations. This pattern of performance is shown in **Fig. 3** and shows differences in mean performance. The performance of the AD and healthy control populations show little overlap, whereas the MCI group performance shows significant overlap with both of the other

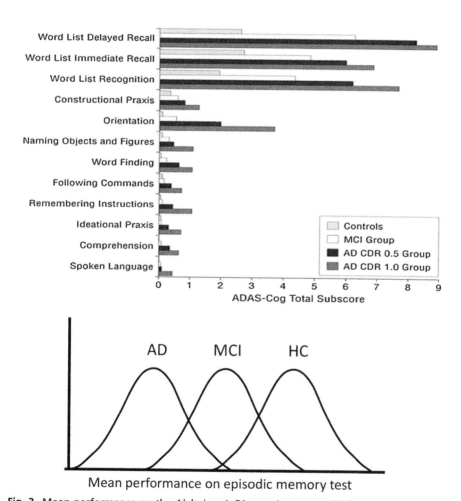

Fig. 3. Mean performance on the Alzheimer's Disease Assessment Scale–Cognitive Subscale subtests. The figure is a hypothetical distribution based on the Grundman 'word list immediate recall' data, showing that whereas the healthy control and AD group distributions differ markedly, the MCI group show significant overlap with both the healthy control and AD group performance. (*Data from* Grundman M, Petersen RC, Ferris SH. Mild cognitive impairment can be distinguished from Alzheimer disease and normal aging for clinical trials. Arch Neurol 2004;61:59–66.)

2 populations. Although the representation is a hypothetical representation of this point, it is nonetheless illustrative of study findings and shows the challenges of dissociating MCI from normal performance.

The need to accurately identify individuals with MCI has received significant impetus from the study designs settled on by those seeking to develop drugs for AD. Until recently, the focus of most AD drug trials has been on patients in the mild-to-moderate stages of the disease, typically those with a baseline MMSE score of between 14 and 26. Various antiamyloid therapies have been targeted at this group of patients, although with exception of AN-1792-201,[9] with little or no evidence of cognitive benefit. Current strategies have been focused on earlier intervention, which has required the identification of patients who have not progressed to AD as determined by diagnostic criteria. A variety of enrichment strategies have been considered, including structural neuroimaging, amyloid load using imaging agents, and cerebrospinal fluid measures of tau and amyloid protein levels. These techniques and methodologies are discussed elsewhere in this issue.

A further enrichment strategy has been the inclusion of cognitive screening measures as further criteria for seeking to recruit appropriate individuals for experimental treatment. Following advice such as that offered by the European Task Force for Alzheimer's Disease,[10] the areas of cognition targeted for screening have tended to be episodic memory, working memory, and executive function. However, the key target area for most studies has been the assessment of episodic memory. This situation is perhaps unsurprising given that often an early warning sign for patients and those around them is noticeable decline in memory function. Episodic memory deficits have been detected using tests of visual memory, often based on paired associative learning (PAL) paradigms requiring study participants to learn to associate visual stimuli with spatial locations (eg Refs.[11,12]). Other computerized tests have included measures of recognition memory in which the study participant is required to view to-be-remembered-items (TBRIs) and later identify the TBRI from one or more foils (ie, stimuli that were not previously presented). Examples of this methodology are the CANTAB Pattern Recognition Test[13] (Cambridge Cognition, Cambridge, UK) and the CDR system Picture Recognition Test (Bracket Global, Goring-on-Thames, UK).[14] There are few paper-and-pencil episodic visual memory tests available for use. Perhaps the best known measures are the Visual Paired Associates learning test, part of the Wechsler Memory Scale,[15] the Brief Visual Memory Test,[16] and the Rey-Osterrieth Complex Figure (ROCF).[17] These tests are often cumbersome to administer and, especially in the case of the ROCF, feature subjective scoring rules. Perhaps because of the paucity of available episodic visual memory tests, investigators of paper-and-pencil episodic memory measures have tended to focus on the assessment of verbal memory. This aspect of cognitive assessment is a component of all of the principal composite measures of cognition (eg, Refs.[1,18]), although often episodic verbal memory has been assessed as a standalone measure. These measures have been shown to function well when used to dissociate AD from the performance of normal, healthy individuals; in the next section, the composition of probably the most widely used screening test for AD is discussed.

CURRENT MODELS OF SCREENING: THE MMSE

Screening measures have traditionally been either composite measures of cognition, such as the MMSE, or tests of single cognitive domains, usually episodic memory. As much of the evidence presented earlier suggests, cognition is not a unitary entity, and given the ubiquity of the MMSE, it makes a good case study of the kinds of composite measures that are used for early AD screening. In the following section, the MMSE is considered in the context of the atoms of cognition described earlier.

The MMSE,[1] originally designed as a brief, bedside measure of global cognition, has been used in several roles. It is commonly used to define patients entering clinical drug trials and is occasionally used as an efficacy measure in these same trials. The scale is weighted heavily toward the measurement of memory, including aspects of orientation to time and place. The orientation component and the immediate and delayed word recall components account for 16 of the possible 30 marks. Attention contributes a further 5 points, with ideational praxis 3 points, confrontation naming 2 points, constructional praxis 1 point, and various aspects of language production and comprehension a further 3 points. In terms of breadth, there is thus some representation of domains such as memory, attention, language, and praxis. However, with as few as 3 words to remember, and just 2 items featuring in the confrontation naming element, the MMSE does not measure these elements in any significant detail. A further significant limitation to its use is the limited versions available. The purpose of the word registration and word recall items is to index episodic memory. The real risk of administering the same 'apple, penny, table' items repeatedly is that these words are rote learned by patients. Thus, the validity of this item is undermined, because in MMSE-naive patients, these items index episodic memory, whereas in others, they index semantic memory. The lack of parallel items extends to all but the orientation items, but then only if the MMSE is administered in a different location on each visit and at a time point when the year, day, date, month, and season have changed. An obvious further limitation is the absence of test elements indexing executive functions.

RECENT REVIEWS OF COGNITIVE SCREENING INSTRUMENTS

The Prevent Alzheimer's Disease 2020 (PAD2020) group have recently overseen a review of the available screening instrumentation. The investigators sought information from instrument investigators and test vendors based on a literature review approach. All parties were invited to submit replies to a questionnaire, responses to which are available on the PAD2020 Web site (http://pad2020.org/). The identified screening instruments included traditional paper-and-pencil measures, but were for the most part computerized measures. Key results of the review were reported in Snyder and colleagues[5] and summary data are reproduced in **Table 4**. Levels of sensitivity and specificity are broadly consistent with those observed with other instruments such as those reported by Lischka and colleagues.[19] Snyder and colleagues received replies from various instrument investigators to the effect that no particular claim was made for the screening usefulness of the instrument. This situation may account for the lack of response from primary investigators who did not participate in the PAD2020 review, such as for the Brief Assessment of Cognition in Schizophrenia (BACS)[20] and Neuropsychological Assessment Battery (NAB),[21] both of which are general cognitive instruments. However, for some of the listed instruments, evidence exists to suggest that they have some usefulness in screening for early dementia. One example of this is the CANTAB system. Evidence has accumulated since work performed by Fowler and colleagues[22] that 1 particular component of the CANTAB system, PAL, could detect individuals who would go on to receive diagnoses of AD 6 months later. This line of research was further developed by Blackwell and colleagues,[11] who determined that the combination of PAL and a confrontation naming test yielded 100% accuracy in detecting who in a sample of individuals would go on to receive a diagnosis of probable AD.

Table 4
Summary of PAD2020 review measures reporting detection sensitivity

System	Reference	Sensitivity	Specificity	Web-Based?	Self-Administered?	Administration Time (min)
Automated Neuropsychological Assessment Metrics	44	93.8	n/a	No	Yes	45
CNS Vital Signs Neuropsychological Assessment Battery	45	54–90	50–95	Yes	Yes	25–30
CogState	12	94	100	Yes	No	20–25
Computer-Administered Neuropsychological Screen for Mild Cognitive Impairment	–	100	100	No	Yes	25–30
Computer Assessment of Mild Cognitive Impairment	46	86	94	No	Yes	20–25
Computerized Self Test	47	96	n/a	Yes	Yes	10–15
Mild Cognitive Impairment Screen	48	95–97	88–99	Yes	No	10
Mindstreams	49	79	95	No	Yes	15–60

SUMMARY AND RECOMMENDATIONS

Earlier in this article, the need was considered to recruit individuals at risk of developing AD so that intervention could be made earlier in the disease process. The limitations of a single, cross-sectional cognitive assessment were also considered, highlighting the fact that initially high-functioning individuals would be missed by a single assessment, because, by definition, such an approach could not capture decline over time. It was further pointed out that traditional paper-and-pencil screening tools were not designed for repeated assessment and so were limited in their usefulness as measures of cognitive change because of practice, learning, and other familiarity effects. A variety of methods exist to determine whether change in an individual's performance is likely caused by measurement error or by a real effect. However, a common factor in the use of these techniques is the importance of test reliability, with measures of temporal reliability featuring in the calculation of key statistics such as the standard error of prediction. Thus, the higher the temporal reliability, or, in the context of other techniques, the smaller the within subject SD, the greater the potential for detecting significant changes. These methods offer a real opportunity of identifying those early in the disease process, not from normative performance, but in light of progressive decline in cognitive performance. However, to maximize the potential of this approach, highly reliable measures of cognition must be used, focused on those domains known to be compromised early in the disease process, specifically episodic memory, working memory, and executive function. A future model of early screening for AD might feature annual cognitive screening, after which performance for the latest visit is compared with that of past visits. Any decline in performance detected would be flagged for further investigation, possibly using technologies discussed elsewhere in this issue.

Given the comments, reviews, and thoughts discussed in this article, it seems helpful to conclude with a review, wish list, and vision of how cognitive screening for the future might look. Good cognitive screening measures have to be based on sound psychometric principles. The articles by Ferris and colleagues[23] and Harrison & Maruff[24] outline many of the key issues; good tests show high levels of reliability, validity, and sensitivity. The usual measure of test-rest reliability remains important, but so too does the issue of stability. A distinction is made between competence (the true level of performance given the best possible circumstances) and performance (the observed test result). Our ambition is to exclude as much error from our measurement as possible and to narrow the gap between competence and performance to a minimum. Robust, reliable, repeatable tests facilitate this process.

A further issue for consideration is the topic of motivation. It is basic good sense that performance is to some degree a function of the participant's motivation. The administration of most paper-and-pencil tests is a dry affair, and many computerized tests are lengthy and boring. This situation seems like an opportunity missed, especially given the extraordinary developments in computer game technology. Computer gaming has affected a variety of disciplines and activities, including games to promote health.[25] However, the innovation and engagement of test participants may not have been exploited to its full potential. Game creators have not just made computer testing fun but have even defined operationally what fun is. The time seems ripe to capitalize on these developments, intuitively it seems reasonable to suppose that interesting and engaging tests induce study participants to try their hardest to do well.

Despite its limitations, cognitive screening possesses several virtues. First, it is typically a relatively cheap screening methodology. The cost of traditional paper-and-pencil assessments, such as the MMSE, typically runs to just a couple of dollars per test. The real cost of these assessments is the time needed to administer and score the test. It is in this context that the cost of computerized assessments should be judged. Two further virtues of cognitive screening are that the measures used are brief and noninvasive.

REFERENCES

1. Folstein MF, Folstein SE, McHugh PR. "Mini-mental state." A practical method for grading the cognitive state of patients for the clinician. J Psychiatr Res 1975; 12(3):189–98.
2. Rentz D, Weintraub S. Neuropsychological detection of early Alzheimer's disease. In: Scinto L, Daffner K, editors. Early diagnosis of Alzheimer's disease. Totowa (NJ): Humana Press; 2000. p. 169–89.
3. Ashford JW. Screening for memory disorder, dementia, and Alzheimer's disease. Aging Health 2008;4(4):399–432.
4. Mendiondo MS, Ashford JW, Kryscio RJ, et al. Designing a Brief Alzheimer Screen (BAS). J Alzheimers Dis 2003;5(5):391–8.
5. Snyder PJ, Jackson CE, Petersen RC, et al. Review article: assessment of cognition in mild cognitive impairment: a comparative study. Alzheimers Dement 2011;7: 338–55.
6. Milner B. Physiologie de l'hippocampe. Les troubles de la mémoire accompagnant des lesions hippocampiques bilatérales. In: Passouant P, editor. Paris: Centre National de la Recherche Scientifique; 1962. p. 257–72.
7. Collie A, Maruff P. An analysis of systems of classifying mild cognitive impairment in older people. Aust N Z J Psychiatry 2002;36:133–40.
8. Grundman M, Petersen RC, Ferris SH. Mild cognitive impairment can be distinguished from Alzheimer disease and normal aging for clinical trials. Arch Neurol 2004;61:59–66.
9. Gilman S, Koller M, Black RS, et al. Clinical effects of Abeta immunization (AN1792) in patients with AD in an interrupted trial. Neurology 2005;64(9):1553–62.
10. Vellas B, Andrieu S, Sampaio C, et al. Disease-modifying trials in Alzheimer's disease: a European task force consensus. Lancet Neurol 2007;6(1):56–62.
11. Blackwell AD, Sahakian BJ, Vesey R, et al. Detecting dementia: novel neuropsychological markers of preclinical Alzheimer's disease. Dement Geriatr Cogn Disord 2004;17(1–2):42–8.
12. Darby D, Pietrzak RH, Fredrickson J, et al. Intra-individual cognitive decline using a brief computerized cognitive screening test. Alzheimers Dement 2012;8(2):95–104.
13. Sahakian BJ, Morris RG, Evenden JL, et al. A comparative-study of visuospatial memory and learning in Alzheimer-type dementia and Parkinson's disease. Brain 1988;111:695–718.
14. Walker MP, Ayre GA, Perry EK, et al. Quantification and characterization of fluctuating cognition in dementia with Lewy bodies and Alzheimer's disease. Dement Geriatr Cogn Disord 2000;11:327–35.
15. Holdnack J, Drozdick L. The Wechsler Memory Scale. San Antonio (TX): Pearson; 2008.
16. Barr W, Morrison C, Zaroff C, et al. Use of the Brief Visuospatial Memory Test-Revised (BVMT-R) in neuropsychological evaluation of epilepsy surgery candidates. Epilepsy Behav 2004;5(2):175–9.
17. Rey A. L'examen psychologique dans les cas d'encéphalopathie traumatique. Les problèmes. Archives de Psychologie 1941;28:215–85.
18. Damian AM, Jacobson SA, Hentz JG, et al. The Montreal Cognitive Assessment and the mini-mental state examination as screening instruments for cognitive

impairment: item analyses and threshold scores. Dement Geriatr Cogn Disord 2011;31:126–31.

19. Lischka AR, Mendelsohn M, Overend T, et al. A systematic review of screening tools for predicting the development of dementia. Can J Aging 2012;31:295–311.

20. Ting C, Rajji TK, Ismail Z, et al. Differentiating the cognitive profile of schizophrenia from that of Alzheimer disease and depression in late life. PLoS One 2010;5(4):e10151.

21. Brown LB, Stern RA, Cahn-Weiner DA, et al. Driving scenes test of the neuropsychological assessment battery (NAB) and on-road driving performance in aging and very mild dementia. Arch Clin Neuropsychol 2005;20:209–15.

22. Fowler KS, Saling MM, Conway EL, et al. Computerized neuropsychological tests in the early detection of dementia: prospective findings. J Int Neuropsychol Soc 1997;3:139–46.

23. Ferris SH, Lucca U, Mohs R, et al. Objective psychometric tests in clinical trials of dementia drugs. Position paper from the International Working Group on Harmonization of Dementia Drug Guidelines. Alzheimer Dis Assoc Disord 1997; 11(Suppl 3):34–8.

24. Harrison JE, Maruff P. Measuring the mind: assessing cognitive change in clinical drug trials. Exp Rev Clin Pharmacol 2008;1(4):471–3.

25. Harrison JE. Fighting Alzheimer's disease: can gaming help cut the costs and save the patient? Presented at Games for Health. Amsterdam; November 5, 2012.

26. Robinson-Whelen S, Storandt M. Immediate and delayed prose recall among normal and demented adults. Arch Neurol 1992;49:32–4.

27. Grober E, Kawas C. Learning and retention in preclinical and early Alzheimer's disease. J Int Neuropsychol Soc 1996;2:12.

28. Locascio JJ, Growden JH, Corkin S. Cognitive test performance in detecting, staging and tracking Alzheimer's disease. Arch Neurol 1995;52:1087–99.

29. Welsh KA, Butters N, Hughes J, et al. Detection of abnormal memory decline in mild cases of Alzheimer's disease using CERAD neuropsychological measures. Arch Neurol 1991;48:278–81.

30. Welsh KA, Butters N, Hughes JP, et al. Detection and staging of dementia in Alzheimer's disease. Arch Neurol 1992;49:448–52.

31. Morris JC, Edland S, Clark C, et al. The Consortium to Establish a Registry for Alzheimer's Disease (CERAD). Part IV. Rates of cognitive change in the longitudinal assessment of probable Alzheimer's disease. Neurology 1993;43:2457–65.

32. Eslinger PJ, Damasio AR. Preserved motor learning in Alzheimer's disease: implications for anatomy and behavior. J Neurosci 1986;6:3006–9.

33. Moscovitch M. Multiple dissociations of function in amnesia. In: Cermak LS, editor. Human memory and amnesia. Hillsdale (NJ): Erlbaum; 1982. p. 337–70.

34. Price BH, Gurvit H, Weintraub S, et al. Neuropsychological patterns and language deficits in twenty consecutive cases of autopsy-confirmed Alzheimer's disease. Arch Neurol 1993;50:931–7.

35. Morris JC, Fulling K. Early Alzheimer's disease. Arch Neurol 1988;45:345–9.

36. Kaszniak AW, Garron DC, Fox J. Differential effects of age and cerebral atrophy upon span of immediate recall and paired associate learning in older patients with suspected dementia. Cortex 1979;15:285–95.

37. Trenerry MR, Crosson B, DeBoe J, et al. Stroop neuropsychological screening test. Odessa (FL): Psychological Assessment Resources; 1989.

38. Benton AL, deS Hamsher K, Varney NR, et al. Contributions to neuropsychological assessment. New York: Oxford University Press; 1983.

39. Reitan RM. Validity of the trail making test as an indication of organic brain damage. Percept Mot Skills 1958;8:271–6.

40. Grady CL, Haxby JV, Horwitz B, et al. A longitudinal study of the early neuropsychological and cerebral metabolic changes in dementia of the Alzheimer's type. J Clin Exp Neuropsychol 1988;10:576–96.

41. Grober E, Lipton RB, Hall C, et al. Memory impairment on free and cued selective reminding predicts dementia. Neurology 2000;54:827–32.

42. Frank RM, Byrne GJ. The clinical utility of the Hopkins Verbal Learning Test as a screening test for mild dementia. Int J Geriatr Psychiatry 2000;15:317–24.

43. Schmidt M. The Rey Auditory Verbal Learning Test. Los Angeles (CA): A Handbook Western Psychological Services; 1996.

44. Levinson D, Reeves D, Watson J, et al. Automated neuropsychological assessment metrics (ANAM) measures of cognitive effects of Alzheimer's disease. Arch Clin Neuropsychol 2005;20:403–8.

45. Gualtieri CT, Johnson LG. Neurocognitive testing supports a broader concept of mild cognitive impairment. Am J Alzheimers Dis Other Demen 2005;20:359–66.

46. Saxton J, Morrow L, Eschman A, et al. Computer assessment of mild cognitive impairment. Postgrad Med 2009;121:177–85.

47. Dougherty JH, Cannon RL, Nicholas CR, et al. The Computerized Self Test: an interactive, Internet accessible cognitive screening test for dementia. J Alzheimers Dis 2010;20:185–95.

48. Shankle WR, Romney AK, Hara J, et al. Method to improve the detection of mild cognitive impairment. Proc Natl Acad Sci U S A 2005;102:4919–24.

49. Simon ES, Goldstein FC, Lah JJ, et al. Computerized cognitive assessment predicts conversion to dementia within two years: interim analysis of a prospective study of MCI. In: International Conference on the Prevention of Dementia. Washington, DC, June 9–12, 2007.

Clinical Trials in Predementia Stages of Alzheimer Disease

Jagan A. Pillai, MBBS, PhD[a],*, Jeffrey L. Cummings, MD, ScD[b]

KEYWORDS

- Preclinical Alzheimer's disease • Prodromal Alzheimer's disease
- Mild cognitive impairment • At-risk population • Clinical trial designs
- Outcome measures • Primary prevention • Secondary prevention

KEY POINTS

- Effective disease-modifying treatments before the onset of clinical dementia are being considered in a new generation of Alzheimer disease (AD) clinical trials.
- The rationale is to intervene before irreversible cognitive deficits.
- New consensus diagnosis of preclinical AD and identifying at-risk asymptomatic individuals are key for reliable targeting of clinical trials.
- Biomarker outcomes in parallel groups are an advantageous model for trial design in this population.
- Novel trial designs, outcome measures, and therapeutic agents are being developed for this population.
- Economic impact of targeting preclinical population is important to consider in developing these clinical trials.
- Integrating clinical, molecular, imaging, and genetic biomarkers and cognitive, functional, and neuropsychiatric variables with small effect sizes over a large trial population to obtain replicable findings are a challenge in clinical trials in preclinical AD.

CLINICAL TRIALS

Dementia is rapidly increasing as the global population ages and is projected to make an enormous impact on all societies. AD is the most common form of dementia, accounting for 60% to 80% of cases. The world Alzheimer Report in 2009 estimated the number of people globally with dementia as 35.6 million, and epidemiologic studies indicate that this number is expected to nearly double every 20 years, to 65.7 million in 2030 and 115.4 million in 2050.[1] The worldwide costs of dementia (US $604 billion in 2010) amount to more than 1% of global gross domestic product.[2]

[a] Lou Ruvo Center for Brain Health, Cleveland Clinic, 9500 Euclid Avenue, Cleveland, OH 44195, USA; [b] Lou Ruvo Center for Brain Health, Cleveland Clinic, 888 West Bonneville Avenue, Las Vegas, NV 89106, USA
* Corresponding author.
E-mail address: pillaij@ccf.org

Med Clin N Am 97 (2013) 439–457
http://dx.doi.org/10.1016/j.mcna.2013.01.002
0025-7125/13/$ – see front matter © 2013 Elsevier Inc. All rights reserved.

medical.theclinics.com

The past 3 decades have seen successes in developing effective symptomatic treatments for AD, but there is still no clinically validated disease-modifying therapy. Recent trials of disease-modifying therapies have been disappointing. Curtailing the impact of AD dementia by effective treatments is an urgent necessity and consensus is growing on the need to shift trials towards predementia subjects to demonstrate efficacy[3] and to treat patients in whom a high level of function can be preserved.

The strides made in understanding the molecular mechanisms of AD in the past 3 decades now shape new disease-modifying treatments that are considered and the means to test their effectiveness. New diagnostic criteria and guidelines for AD by the International Working Group (IWG)[4,5] and by the National Institute on Aging and the Alzheimer's Association, in 2011, include molecular and imaging biomarkers developed recently.[6–9] These criteria, which specify preclinical AD as a separate diagnostic entity, are expected to help in shifting the focus of treatments to early stages of the disease. Failed treatment trials attempting to reduce brain amyloid in AD dementia have suggested the importance of intervening early in the AD process.[10] With the criteria for preclinical AD in place, a new generation of disease modifiers can be effectively tested at early stages of AD. They will focus on biologic changes occurring in the disease process before irreversible neuropathologic damage. This may halt the progression of the disease before significant neural damage, help preserve higher levels of function, or delay development of clinical milestones of the disease. Similar approaches have been effective in other chronic diseases, including diabetes and cardiovascular diseases.

Therapeutic intervention, when planned early in the disease process among asymptomatic individuals, before clinical symptoms and biologic markers are observed, is termed, *primary prevention*; in secondary prevention, the focus is asymptomatic individuals with biologic evidence of underlying disease; tertiary prevention aims at slowing or deferring progression of mild symptoms of symptomatic individuals. In this sense, the Anti-Amyloid Treatment in Asymptomatic Alzheimer's Disease (A4) trial is secondary prevention (**Fig. 1**).

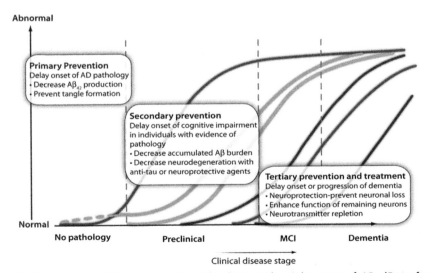

Fig. 1. Testing the right target and the right drug at the right stage of AD. (*Data from* Sperling RA, Jack CR Jr, Aisen PS. Testing the right target and right drug at the right stage. Sci Transl Med 2011;3:111–33.)

With regard to AD primary prevention trials, asymptomatic individuals consist of 3 subgroups: (1) individuals who will never develop AD, (2) those who will eventually develop AD but do not yet show the pathologic hallmarks, and (3) those who have the disease present in nascent form but have yet to manifest clinical changes.[11,12] In order to have effective primary prevention trials, ways to enrich the clinical trial population with individuals in the 2nd and 3rd subgroups have to be actively sought. Enrichment is intended to either maximize the chance of progression to the next stage of AD, which is a dichotomous outcome, or maximize the degree of progression, which is a continuous outcome.[13] Three general approaches to constructing populations for primary prevention trials can be considered: (1) inclusion of all individuals older than a specific age, using age as the only indicator of risk; (2) inclusion of persons with an elevated risk profile based on epidemiologic factors known to predispose to AD in addition to age (eg, history of hypertension or presence of apolipoprotein E [APOE] 4 allele; and (3) identification of at-risk individuals through the use of biomarkers that change in anticipation of clinical decline (eg, amyloid imaging).[12]

In tertiary AD prevention trials, the predementia subjects are already expected to show early neuropathologic changes of AD. Successful interventions in secondary AD prevention are expected to decrease the burden of neuropathology or delay its accrual and influence the biomarkers, denoting a deferral or arrest in the disease process with a corresponding impact on progression of clinical symptoms. Cognitive tests with a good signal-to-noise profile (measure of sensitivity to decline, such as the mean–to–standard deviation ratio) in tracking change over time are crucial in secondary prevention trials, so that change over time in individual subjects is not lost in the variance in cognitive status that is common in any population. Because many secondary prevention AD trials focus on targeting the amyloid burden, identifying amyloid-positive but cognitively normal subjects (AD endophenotype) becomes challenging. It is not efficient to screen an entire population with amyloid imaging or a lumbar puncture for cerebrospinal fluid (CSF) amyloid to identify eligible individuals with brain amyloidosis. Substitute markers, such as age and APOE genotype, are useful predictors of the likelihood of significant amyloid accumulation and used to screen individuals, followed by more detailed amyloid testing.[14]

TRIALS WITH ASYMPTOMATIC INDIVIDUALS

Autosomal dominant AD provides a good model to study disease progression and test primary prevention interventions in as-yet asymptomatic persons. In autosomal dominant AD, penetrance is complete; both who will develop the disease (mutation carriers) and when clinical onset is to be expected (consistent within families) are predictable. Large retrospectively and prospectively assessed cohorts of descendants with familial AD have been tracked to document early symptoms.[15,16] Secondary prevention trials can be focused on specific biomarkers and neuropsychological measures. Down syndrome has also been proposed as a model to study early stage of AD as it is accompanied by neuropathologic features of AD.[17] In these studies, enrichment based on comparing mutation carriers with noncarriers is an excellent way to optimize a clinical outcome for measuring progression over time.[13]

Trials of subjects with inherited or familial AD are not without challenges and it is difficult to know how to extrapolate these findings to sporadic AD. Fewer than 3% of patients with AD have mutations of the amyloid precursor protein, presenilin 1 (PS1), or presenilin 2 (PS2) genes. These mutations account for most cases of familial AD.[18–20] Not all individuals who develop familial AD follow the same clinical trajectory. There is significant phenotypic heterogeneity observed between different genetic mutations associated with familial AD and they cannot be lumped together with regard to clinical progression.[21] Biomarker abnormalities are present in presymptomatic familial AD but their significance and interpretation require correlation with clinical stage of disease and a subject's cognitive profile.[21–23] Objective cognitive changes are observed several years before clinically meaningful symptoms in many familial AD patients.[16] Anxiety may play a role in these subjective symptoms, or it may be that standard neuropsychological tests are not sensitive enough to detect the earliest deficits in highly educated participants.[20] Finding appropriate markers of early cognitive processing changes by multimodal imaging for tracking effectiveness of therapeutic interventions is one way to pursue overcoming this problem. Due to the younger age of onset in familial AD, patients in these cohorts often have less comorbid illness and less use of concomitant medications. These factors could influence the symptoms and the course of clinical progression compared with older individuals with more comorbidities. Therapeutic interventions in predementia populations are targeted to biologic mechanisms of AD pathology, and there are substantial differences between familial AD and sporadic AD (**Table 1**). The γ-secretase enzyme, important in amyloid-β (Aβ) production, is altered by PS1 and PS2 mutations and there is increased production of amyloid (AB42) compared with sporadic AD. These factors might influence therapeutic interventions targeted to amyloid clearance and may make it harder to generalize clinical trial results from familial to sporadic AD.

In addition to familial AD, cognitively normal people with a high risk of developing AD dementia include carriers of 2 copies of the *APOE* ε4 allele.[24] These subjects have been shown to have imaging changes, including hippocampal,[25] whole-brain,[26] and medial temporal lobe cortical atrophy[27]; functional imaging changes, such as regional changes on task-activated functional MRI,[28] connectivity changes,[29] and decrease of posterior cingulate activity measured by fluorodeoxyglucose–positron emission tomography (FDG-PET)[30]; and higher fibrillar Aβ burden.[31] Cognitively normal *APOE* ε4 carriers have low $A\beta_{42}$ levels and high total-tau and phospho-tau levels in CSF. These biomarkers could be used to evaluate preclinical AD in cognitively normal late–middle-aged *APOE* ε4 homozygotes or heterozygotes for inclusion in primary or secondary prevention trials.[31]

Although familial AD involves less than 3% of AD, a recent study suggests that rare variants of familial AD increase risk for late-onset sporadic AD.[32] One small (6 subjects) open-label prevention trial with β-hydroxy-β-methylglutaryl–CoA reductase inhibitor as therapeutic intervention in familial AD has been completed.[33] A significantly larger

Table 1
Differences between autosommal dominant and sporadic AD

Autosomal Dominant AD	Sporadic AD
γ-Secretase mutations	No γ-secretase alterations
Increased Aβ production	Decreased Aβ clearance
Young onset	Older age onset
Comorbidity limited	Comorbidity common
Few concomitant medications	Concomitant medications common
Familial expectations	Limited inheritance expectations
Behavioral features more common	Behavioral features less common
More aphasia	Less aphasia
More rapid progression	Slower progression
Striatal amyloid deposition	No/limited striatal amyloid deposition

undertaking is the Dominantly Inherited Alzheimer Network (DIAN), a worldwide network of centers studying autosomal-dominant AD. DIAN has determined the timing and order of changes in autosomal-dominant AD in a large cohort with the disease. The study found that amyloid changes begin in the brain at least 2 decades before the estimated onset of clinical symptoms.[16] If the nature and sequence of brain changes in autosomal dominant AD is generalizable to sporadic AD, targeting of Aβ earlier in the course of the disease may provide better clinical outcomes than the treatment of mild to moderate dementia involving patients with substantial neuronal and synaptic loss. Based on this rationale, DIAN therapeutic trials unit has recently started a 2-year study of the effects of 3 AD drugs in the preclinical population: gantenerumab, solanezumab (amyloid-binding immunomodulating agents), and LY2886721 (β-secretase inhibitor) compared with a shared placebo group. Each drug arm will enroll 80 people, assigning noncarriers to placebo, to maintain genetic status blinding, and randomizing mutation carriers to drug versus placebo in a 3-to-1 ratio. The first phase will last 2 years, at which point drugs that met primary aims of affecting any downstream biomarkers (tau and phospho-tau proteins in the CSF, alterations in functional brain imaging, and brain atrophy and cortical thinning in MRI) of neurodegeneration would be considered for longer-term cognitive endpoint studies.

In linkage disequilibrium with *APOE* gene is the AD susceptibility locus within the translocase of outer mitochondrial membrane 40 homolog (TOMM40) gene. An association between different lengths—short, long, and very long—of a poly-T locus in TOMM40 has been reported with ages of AD onset.[34] Long alleles of this locus were nearly always linked to *APOE* ε4 and associated with greater disease risk. Thus, the TOMM40 poly-T locus and *APOE* genotype may differentiate subjects at higher and lower age-dependent risk of developing mild cognitive impairment (MCI) due to AD and subsequently AD dementia. The expression of *APOE* is further transcriptionally regulated by the ligand-activated nuclear receptor, peroxisome proliferator–activated receptor γ (PPARγ). This has been of interest in a new therapeutic avenue for asymptomatic gene-positive individuals who carry the TOMM40 gene. A subject enrichment algorithm based on this rationale is being developed for use in a preclinical AD trail by a Takeda/Zinfandel clinical trial consortium for a therapeutic trail of the PPARγ agonist, pioglitazone. PPARγ agonists play critical roles in energy metabolism due to their direct effects on mitochondrial function and ATP production. The effects of PPARγ agonists on mitochondrial structure and function may be the basis of their beneficial effects on cognition in AD subjects. The effectiveness of pioglitazone in preventing future onset of cognitive decline in asymptomatic subjects is to be tested.

A large study involving familial AD is the Alzheimer Prevention Initiative (API). Cognitively normal PS1 E280A mutation carriers, at least 35 years of age (ie, within 10 years of the carriers' estimated median age at clinical onset), from the world's largest known early-onset AD kindred, located in Antioquia, Colombia, will be randomized to active treatment or placebo with the noncarriers assigned only to placebo with changes in amyloid PET, FDG-PET, volumetric MRI, CSF, and cognitive scores as endpoints.[31,35] Crenezumab, a monoclonal antibody, will be the interventional agent.

A trial in asymptomatic subjects is proposed by the Alzheimer's Disease Cooperative Study (ADCS), the A4 trial.[10] The A4 trial aims to study the impact of anti-Aβ amyloid treatment on downstream markers of neurodegeneration (tau and phospho-tau proteins in the CSF, alterations in functional brain imaging, and brain atrophy and cortical thinning) and explore whether there is a critical window for anti-Aβ amyloid therapy within the preclinical stages of AD. It also aims to develop more sensitive outcome measures to improve the efficiency of future secondary prevention trials.

It plans to recruit older subjects (>70 years) who are cognitively normal but have a positive amyloid PET and compare an antiamyloid drug against a placebo in approximately 1000 people for 3 years of double-blind treatment.

TRIALS WITH PRODROMAL AD POPULATIONS

Prodromal AD, as described by the International Working Group, refers to the early symptomatic, predementia phase of AD in which (1) clinical symptoms, including episodic memory loss of the hippocampal type (characterized by a free recall deficit on testing not normalized with cueing), are present but not sufficiently severe to affect activities of daily living (ADL) and do not warrant a diagnosis of dementia and in which (2) biomarker evidence from CSF or imaging is supportive of the presence of AD pathologic changes.[4,5] Rather than requiring identification of functional impairments that allow a distinction between MCI and dementia, prodromal AD relies on a combination of patient-reported or informant-reported and cognitive test–based evidence of progressive change in memory and at least 1 of several imaging or CSF biomarkers that have been associated with an AD diagnosis.

This working definition of prodromal AD reduces the heterogeneity of MCI useful for therapeutic trials targeting biologic pathways of AD. Some models of AD disease progression have proposed that future clinical trials for prodromal AD could be made more efficient by requiring a CSF $A\beta_{1-42}$ biomarker.[36,37] Recent clinical trials have used prodromal AD populations, as in the multicenter, randomized, double-blind, placebo-controlled, parallel-group study to evaluate the effect of gantenerumab (RO4909832).[38] These inclusion criteria are also used in safety and tolerability studies of avagacestat and BIIB037. There are critiques that the requirement of biomarker-positive patients would most likely not result in more efficient clinical trials (if effect size is assumed proportional to the signal-to-noise ratio of the Alzheimer Disease Assessment Scale–cognitive subscale [ADAS-cog]) and that trials would take longer to recruit because fewer patients would be available.[39] Use of prodromal AD as an entry criterion may address the problem in MCI trials of regression to the mean, stemming from using a clinical outcome (memory decline) to identify subjects for a study and a related clinical outcome (memory decline) to follow those same subjects over time.[40]

TRIALS WITH MILD COGNITIVE IMPAIRMENT

Individuals with MCI show evidence of lower performance in one or more cognitive domains that is greater than expected for patient age and educational background. A decline in performance is also often evident over time.[6] Pathologic investigation reveals that patients with prospectively diagnosed MCI who die before advancing to diagnosable Alzheimer-type dementia have neuropathologic changes of the Alzheimer type in excess of those found in normal controls.[41–44] Despite this high correlation between the clinical diagnosis of MCI and underlying neuropathologic changes consistent with early AD, long-term follow-up study of patients diagnosed with MCI suggests that nearly one-third develop non-AD primary pathologic abnormalities.[45] MCI may, therefore, be regarded as a syndrome that is often (but not always) associated with Alzheimer pathology and has variable outcomes. Longitudinal studies of well-characterized MCI patients show progression or conversion of MCI to AD dementia in the range of 10% to 15% per year.[46,47] The different rate of progression to dementia in each treatment arm serves as the rationale for a clinical trial paradigm that compares therapeutic benefit between a therapeutic agent and placebo over the course of time, a survival-type analysis.

The first generation of MCI trials identified several implementation challenges. Operationalization of MCI versus dementia diagnosis has been problematic even by expert panels and the diagnostic accuracy of MCI criteria used in different MCI trials has varied.[48] The progression from MCI to dementia is indolent, and it is challenging to assign a specific time to conversion even with the use of expert consensus review of each case. The rate of progression from MCI to AD varies greatly among the trials, from a high of 16% per year (ADCS trial of donepezil, vitamin E, or placebo) to a low of 4% to 5% per year (studies of rivastigmine and rofecoxib).[49–51] This variability in progression rate was most likely related to differences in enrollment criteria and may also reflect intrastudy variability in the frequency of APOE ε4 genotype, depression, and the choice of neuropsychological variables used to track progression.[12] A continuous outcome analysis, such as drug-placebo differences in change in the Clinical Dementia Rating (CDR) scale, may be more meaningful.[52] In addition, floor effects on memory and differences in non-memory features among subjects may influence the ability to capture the rate of clinical progression.[12]

The use of AD biomarkers in MCI could serve to enrich trials with patients who have an early symptomatic form of AD and help overcome some of the challenges of the first generation of MCI clinical trials. They form a definite diagnostic category of MCI due to AD. Most longitudinal studies show higher rates of progression from MCI to AD in individuals with the APOE ε4 genotype. Furthermore, MRI measures, especially medial temporal lobe atrophy, may be used as inclusion measures or surrogate outcomes.[53,54] Stratification of an MCI population into groups that do and do not progress to dementia using CSF measurement of tau and $A\beta_{42}$ have also been shown by 2 independent groups.[55,56] Recent clinical trials have used amyloid imaging and/or CSF $A\beta_{1-42}$ as biomarkers. Even though these biomarkers can help select subjects with MCI who are likely to progress within a defined time interval, it remains possible that this approach risks excluding patients who have AD but progress at different rates.

Despite the caveats, new amyloid markers (imaging and CSF measures) have an advantage for trials of disease-modifying therapeutic strategies that target amyloid synthesis or clearance from the brain. Selection of subjects with biomarker evidence of amyloid accumulation is expected to help enroll an enriched population that is most likely to demonstrate the benefits of an amyloid clearance strategy. The use of several predictor variables for AD (age, episodic memory deficit, and APOE) and biomarkers as entry criteria for a clinical trial brings the MCI due to AD approach close to the prodromal AD definition. Within the AD phenotype, differences in age of onset and in clinical and behavioral symptoms[57] in brain regions of neuropathologic burden[58] and trajectories of clinical progression[59] are recognized. Pharmacologic trials have indicated different AD subtypes with differing responses to specific pharmacotherapies.[60,61] As these differences are better understood at a clinicopathologic-molecular level, additional stratification of AD subjects for effective therapeutic targets will be increasingly meaningful.

DESIGNS FOR CLINICAL TRIALS OF ASYMPTOMATIC POPULATIONS

The randomized controlled clinical trial (RCT) is the gold standard for testing the efficacy of various types of intervention. Challenges in designing RCTs for asymptomatic populations include (1) convincing normal subjects to undergo therapeutic intervention and the risk it entails; (2) the large number of asymptomatic subjects needed to detect a significant reduction in the occurrence of AD over 5 years; (3) long duration of study and high attrition rates; (4) natural heterogeneity in rate of AD progression among individuals when the signal-to-noise ratio is small; (5) education level and demographic factors found consistently different in AD trial populations versus AD subjects in the community, limiting generalization of trial results; (6) choosing appropriate surrogate endpoints, including biomarker changes, to help make the studies more tractable and of shorter duration; and (7) the average progression in this preclinical disease, which is not always clinically relevant, and its importance for the subjects themselves, which may depend on social, educational, and cultural factors.

For asymptomatic/preclinical populations, specific types of RCTs could be used to answer the questions of interest or to gather useful information. Parallel-group RCT is the design of choice for AD therapeutic trials in asymptomatic subjects. Two interventions are given, with one group receiving the medication of interest while another group receives the placebo. The progressive decline over time that almost always occurs with AD and with normal aging eliminates the possibility of a crossover design, because one of the key requirements of a crossover design is that patients are identical at the beginning of both phases.

Delay to milestone designs have been used in MCI clinical trials where time to AD dementia is used as a dichotomous endpoint in a survival analysis.[62,63] As clinical and pathologic heterogeneity within the AD phenotype is increasingly recognized, within-arm stratification of asymptomatic subjects based on these differences (genetic variants and rate of change in regional imaging markers of cognitive processing) could help detect meaningful therapeutic effectiveness that may be missed in a simpler design. This could also be advantageous as delay to fixed milestones (such as dementia) could entail long durations of follow-up that are difficult to implement in the preclinical population. This approach shows promise for use in preclinical AD trials but the test-retest reliability of detecting early cognitive changes is unclear.

Adaptive trial designs based on bayesian probability are of increasing interest in asymptomatic populations. An adaptive design allows modifications to be made to trial and/or statistical procedures of ongoing clinical trials. They are flexible and efficient in the early and late phases of clinical development. It is a concern that the patient population after the adaptations could deviate from the original target patient population and, consequently, the overall type I error (to erroneously claim efficacy for an ineffective drug) rate may not be controlled.[64]

OUTCOMES FOR CLINICAL TRIALS FOR PREDEMENTIA/PRODROMAL AD

Outcome measures in prodromal populations are more challenging than in AD dementia populations because the decline that is observed in predementia populations is less. Composite quantitative outcomes may be more likely to detect reliable change than a single primary outcome measure. Although biomarkers are better than clinical outcomes for identifying individuals in the predementia stages of AD, relying exclusively on biomarkers has the risk that a treatment effect on a biomarker may not translate into a treatment effect on a clinical outcome. There is a further risk of missing any symptomatic effect different from a disease modifying effect.[40] Due to the intrinsic variability in cognitive testing, a combination of biomarkers and cognitive scales may be a more useful outcome.

A widely used primary outcome measure in AD clinical trials is the ADAS-cog.[65,66] The ADAS-cog yields a single score but measures several domains of cognition, including, recall, recognition, orientation, language comprehension, naming, and praxis. It lacks measures of attention, planning, working memory, and executive function.[65] Since its inception more than 2 decades ago, it has been used extensively in dementia clinical trials and its properties are well understood. For use in the predementia population, it faces significant challenges because there is a curvilinear relationship between disease severity and rate of change on the ADAS-cog. In mild to moderate AD, more than half of the ADAS-cog components have substantial percentages of people (often >75%) scoring either 0 or 1, implying few or no problems in cognitive performance in these domains.[67] Differential weighting of ADAS-cog items is an option to improve sensitivity in measuring progression over time in MCI subjects and has been shown to perform better than any single MRI measure in predicting progression from MCI to AD dementia.[68]

The neuropsychological test battery (NTB) is a panel of 6 validated, cognitive tests, yielding 9 measures of memory and/or executive function commonly involved in AD.[69,70] Preliminary observations suggest that the NTB has an advantage over ADAS-cog in that it shows similar decline in patients with mild (high baseline Mini-Mental State Examination score, 21–26) and moderate (low baseline Mini-Mental State Examination score, 15–20). Annual rate of change on a cognitive scale and its variance are among the key elements used in sample size determinations and study duration decisions for clinical trials. Disease-modifying treatment trials, in which subjects with mild AD are more likely to be enrolled, may need a smaller number of subjects to detect a change from baseline for the treatment when using NTB compared with ADAS-cog because NTB seems to have a more linear relationship between disease severity and rate of change. More trial experience with the NTB is needed to fully establish its performance characteristics.

ADL measures can be primary or secondary outcomes in US regulation trials and are required by the European Medicines Agency for approval of antidementia medications in Europe. Patients with MCI perform significantly poorer than age-matched and gender-matched cognitively unimpaired controls on informant interviews of complex ADL. And unlike AD dementia, there is a strong correlation between patient level of cognitive performance and ability to carry out everyday tasks in MCI.[71] Changes in ADL performance and functional deterioration occur in a hierarchical order, affecting more complex followed by simpler activities; functional rating scales are, therefore, useful in grading the severity of functional disabilities. The ADCS MCI-ADL scale, a modification of the ADCS-ADL scale, is designed to optimize sensitivity to impairments in instrumental activities that may occur in MCI and may be more relevant to the predementia/prodromal AD population.[72] The ADL–Prevention Instrument was developed by the ADCS for AD prevention trials. It comprises 15 ADL and 5 physical function questions where an ADL change during a trial could trigger detailed evaluation or serve as an outcome measure. The ADL–Prevention Instrument, obtained from either self-report or informants, discriminated between subjects rated as CDR 0 and CDR 0.5.[73]

The Disability Assessment for Dementia (DAD) scale is a caregiver-based interview that uses a 46-item questionnaire to evaluate instrumental and basic ADL in dementia[74]; approximately 25% of individuals with mild to moderate AD are rated as either unchanged or improved at 1 year[75] and may be less sensitive in preclinical AD populations.

The Alzheimer's Disease Functional Assessment of Change Scale (ADFACS) is a 16-item functional assessment instrument based on both basic ADL and instrumental ADL that has been used in clinical trials of AD dementia.[76] Its use in preclinical AD has not been reported.

Asymptomatic subjects in clinical trials are expected to be fully independent in their functional abilities, and the magnitude of benefit on functional measures that is clinically meaningful in this population is different from that in MCI subjects. One way the variability between patients has been approached has been to define an amount of clinically meaningful change prospectively for each patient and then use that definition to establish an endpoint in a survival analysis.[76,77] This approach shows promise for use in preclinical AD trials.

An important primary outcome measure, according to Food and Drug Administration (FDA) guidelines, is a clinician's global assessment. FDA recommendations for dementia treatments state that (1) a clinically useful drug must have a clinical effect, not only a cognitive one, and (2) the clinical effectiveness of new treatments should be apparent to experienced clinicians.[78] The judgment as to whether a patient improved or worsened or was unchanged is made by a clinician who is blinded to the scores from the cognitive tests of the primary outcome measure. There are 2 types of global judgment–based methods, specified and unspecified. The CDR Scale Sum of Boxes (CDR-SB) is an operationalized measure where a clinician performs specified tests and asks specific questions whereas the Clinical Global Impression of Change plus Caregiver Input (CGIC+) is a checklist measure with less standardization.[79]

The CDR-SB is a well-validated instrument that has been in use for more than 20 years in clinical trials of AD and MCI. The CDR assesses 3 domains of cognition (memory, orientation, and judgment/problem solving) and 3 domains of function (community affairs, home/hobbies, and personal care) and can be summed to assess both cognitive and functional domains of AD disability.[52] The mean scores decline nearly linearly across different severities of AD in the 2-year Alzheimer's Disease Neuroimaging Initiative (ADNI) study; CDR-SB cognitive and functional subscales contribute equally to total scores at both very mild (early) and mild stages of the disease.[80] These factors make it an attractive instrument to track preclinical AD. In both MCI and cognitively normal subjects, baseline positive amyloid imaging scans were associated with greater clinical worsening on the CDR-SB and the ADAS-cog.[81] CDR-SB seems to provide a readily available and easily applicable global assessment of cognitive and functional ability and is significantly associated with the severity of amyloid burden[81] and metabolic deficits in patients with AD.[82]

The ADCS–Clinical Global Impression of Change (ADCS-CGIC) represents a validated and straightforward approach to a clinician's global rating using interviews of both the patient and caregiver.[83] There are also self-rated and study partner–rated versions available to be completed at home with minimal supervision in AD prevention trials.

The Clinician's Interview-Based Impression of Change–Plus (CIBIC+) is among the most widely used global metric of change in dementia clinical trials.[79] It uses Likert scales, recording disease severity and changes during and/or at the end of treatment. It has written accounts summarizing semistructured interviews evaluating behavior, cognition, and function. There is considerable skepticism in the literature about the methodology and inter-rater reliability of the scale.[79,84] Qualitative analyses of the CIBIC+ revealed inconsistencies in the format, content, referents, data collection, and clinicians' model of what represents a treatment effect.[84]

The Mail-In Cognitive Function Screening Instrument (MCFSI) was developed for the ADCS Prevention Instrument Project to evaluate whether a brief mail-in screening tool can be used as a specific and sensitive trigger for a diagnostic evaluation in the course of an AD prevention trial. The MCFSI consists of 2 similar sets of 14 questions mailed separately to the subject and the study partner, who are asked to complete them independently. The questions relate to the decline in function over the past year. MCFSI captures information related to cognitive and functional status in nondemented elderly individuals.[85]

Neuropsychiatric symptoms are common in AD but are expected to be absent in asymptomatic individuals and rare in preclinical AD.[86,87] In AD dementia clinical trials, behavioral changes have been a secondary outcome. Assessment of behavioral symptoms is important because impairments can compromise both cognitive and functional abilities. The Neuropsychiatric Inventory (NPI) is the standard scale used in most AD dementia clinical trials. The NPI evaluates the frequency and severity of 10 neuropsychiatric disturbances that occur frequently in dementia: agitation, irritability, anxiety, dysphoria, hallucinations, delusions, apathy, euphoria, disinhibition, and aberrant motor behavior.[88] At baseline, neuropsychiatric symptoms are expected to be absent or uncommon in preclinical AD and are expected to become more frequent in the course of AD. The NPI can be a secondary endpoint or used as part of a composite score in evaluating disease-modifying therapies in preclinical AD populations.

The economic impact of time spent by the primary caregiver supervising the patient and assisting with ADL can be measured quantitatively by the Resource Utilization in Dementia (RUD) instrument. The RUD scale is completed by caregivers and captures data on the use of social services, frequency and duration of hospitalizations, unscheduled contacts with health care professionals, use of concomitant medications by both caregiver and patient, amount of time a caregiver spends caring for the patient and missing work, and patients' use of study medication. The RUD Lite is an abbreviated instrument, developed for cost-effectiveness studies in dementia care.[89–92]

The world population is aging rapidly and society is facing increasing associated costs, whereas health systems face finite budgets. As a result, payers require or at least consider phase III cost-effectiveness data (in addition to safety and efficacy data) for drug and reimbursement. This may increase the risks and costs of drug development in asymptomatic drug trials where no clinically relevant abnormality has yet occurred in subjects being considered. New strategies to generate these key data are needed.[93]

AGENTS TO BE CONSIDERED FOR PREDEMENTIA TRIALS

Disease-modifying agents in preclinical AD (Individuals who have evidence of early AD pathological changes but do not meet clinical criteria for MCI or dementia) attempt to prevent the development of AD-related pathologic changes and/or alter disease progression. Pharmaceutical companies have begun phase II testing of therapeutic agents in patients who are in the predementia stage of AD (**Box 1**). The categories of agents relevant to predementia AD are the same as those of AD dementia. Staging of agents and combination therapies may evolve as data accrues.

IMPLEMENTING TRIALS IN PRECLINICAL AD
Recruitment and Retention

There are many challenges to effective recruitment and retention of participants in predementia AD trials. The follow-up period of 2 to 3 years that is commonly used in first-generation MCI studies may be short because it may take up to 10 years before subjects with preclinical AD progress to AD-type dementia. Studies that are too long require too many visits or that target enrollments of populations too difficult to recruit are in danger of slow or inadequate enrollment. Additional challenges are to ensure that study participants have AD pathology and are representative of the population in the wider community with AD. Availability of amyloid PET and CSF testing is an important requirement for centers participating in predmentia trials. These procedures increase the costs of such trials (both patient burden and financial cost). Once recruited, it is important that subjects complete the study. A variety of factors within a trial may identify patients who will drop out before study completion.

Box 1
Categories of medications to be considered for treatment of predementia population

Neurotransmitter therapies
- Cholinergic
- Nicotinergic
- Serotonergic
- Cannabinoid
- Histaminergic
- Phosphodiesterase inhibition

Protein-related therapies
- Antiamyloid
- Tau related
- TDP-43 related

Cellular processes
- Anti-inflammatory
- Antioxidant
- Mitochondrial
- Peroxisome proliferator–activated receptor (PPAR) agonists
- Synaptic maintenance
- Myelin maintenance

Restoration
- Growth factors
- Stem cells
- Synaptic enhancement

Characteristics of participants who were likely to drop out in previous RCTs include race other than white, less than high school education, and being unmarried (that is, having an adult child or child-in-law as a study partner). Biases in retention make it challenging to generalize results to the general population.

Sites

The most straightforward approach to improving the rate of enrollment is to increase the number of AD trial sites. AD trials have become increasingly global, enrolling from multiple countries and continents within single studies. Global studies have concerns in terms of heterogeneity of the pool of participants and differences in individual regulatory agencies and practices of clinical trial approval in clinically normal subject populations.[94]

Analyses suggest that all sites vary in important ways. Participants recruited to commercial trial sites (as opposed to academic sites) were at increased risk to drop out, influencing the quality of data collected.[95] To plan the recruitment of adequate subject populations for these trials, it is necessary to better understand the pool of eligible patients and the capabilities of the sites for sustained and meaningful engagement with their preclinical AD populations.

Number of Patients

It has been estimated that between 3000 and 6000 subjects are required to detect a 30% reduction in the occurrence of AD over 5 years, assuming a 5% to 10% cumulative incidence of the disease in a preventive study.[96] Recruiting and returning such large numbers of subjects require new and innovative strategies. Stratification of patients based on differences in biomarkers predicting progression and selecting appropriate and meaningful measures of change to be detected are crucial to help reduce the number of subjects involved, toward which there is ongoing research effort.

Social media may provide an avenue to specifically target adult children caregivers. The more reasons a person has for being in a trial, the more likely he or she is to enroll and, over time, stay in a trial. This makes it important to have community-wide engagement and educating regarding the occurrence of the AD disease process decades before symptoms appear.

Screen Failures

The cost of drug development has gone up in part due to the higher costs associated with enrolling subjects at clinical investigative sites. Screen failure is a metric that reveals how well personnel can identify subjects that are expected to qualify and if they understand the enrollment criteria for that study. The financial impact of screen failures in clinical trials is determined by 2 factors: cost per failure and probability of occurrence. If the cost of a failure is nominal, then the burden of even high-probability events may be negligible. If the cost of a failure is high, however, then even a low probability of failure may give pause, and the question of who pays for screen failures—sponsor or investigative site—becomes important.[97] In predementia trials, an additional source of screen failure is patients with normal Aβ biomarkers but who have abnormal levels of neurodegeneration, suspected non-Alzheimer pathophysiology (sNAP). Such patients will have the entire costly screening assessment but may not be entered into the trial.[98]

COMMENT AND SUMMARY

The field of AD therapeutics, after a spate of recent disease-modifying trial failures, is regrouping. New research has shed some light into possible reasons for lack of efficacy. Recent studies in familial AD suggest that the earliest changes start even 20 years before the MCI stage and have prompted interest in preclinical and prodromal AD populations for therapeutic interventions. Advances in biomarkers to track the changes in AD over time, even when there are no obvious clinical symptoms, are crucial in making this shift.

Initiatives, such as the Alzheimer's Disease Neuroimaging Initiative (ADNI),[99] have provided the means to begin mapping the interrelationships among biomarkers and cognitive and clinical disease features, facilitating early AD diagnostic efforts as well as other aspects of trial design. Studies have provided information that can be used for furthering trial design in the early, preclinical AD population.

These challenges are in extrapolating biomarker and AD progression results from specialized populations, such as ADNI (which is homogenous in terms of high education, white race, and high socioeconomic status) or familial AD (where a rare mutation is present), to asymptomatic subjects in the general population. Addressing these complex issues promises to lead to new therapies that will prevent or defer the onset of cognitive impairment or keep patients functioning at nearly asymptomatic levels.

These therapies will dramatically reduce the morbidity of AD and improve quality of life for millions of older people.

REFERENCES

1. Alzheimer's Disease International. World Alzheimer Report 2009. [Accessed on February 06, 2013]. Available at: http://www.alz.co.uk/research/files/World%20Alzheimer%20Report.pdf.
2. Alzheimer's Disease International. World Alzheimer Report 2011.[Accessed on February 06, 2013]. Available at: http://www.alz.co.uk/research/files/World%20Alzheimer%20Report.pdf.
3. Aisen PS. Clinical trial methodologies for disease-modifying therapeutic approaches. Neurobiol Aging 2011;32(Suppl 1):S64–6.
4. Dubois B, Feldman HH, Jacova C, et al. Revising the definition of Alzheimer's disease: a new lexicon. Lancet Neurol 2010;9(11):1118–27.
5. Dubois B, Feldman HH, Jacova C, et al. Research criteria for the diagnosis of Alzheimer's disease: revising the NINCDS-ADRDA criteria. Lancet Neurol 2007; 6(8):734–46.
6. Albert MS, DeKosky ST, Dickson D, et al. The diagnosis of mild cognitive impairment due to Alzheimer's disease: recommendations from the National Institute on Aging–Alzheimer's Association workgroups on diagnostic guidelines for Alzheimer's disease. Alzheimers Dement 2011;7(3):270–9.
7. Jack CR, Albert MS, Knopman DS, et al. Introduction to the recommendations from the National Institute on Aging–Alzheimer's Association workgroups on diagnostic guidelines for Alzheimer's disease. Alzheimers Dement 2011;7(3):257–62.
8. McKhann GM, Knopman DS, Chertkow H, et al. The diagnosis of dementia due to Alzheimer's disease: recommendations from the National Institute on Aging–Alzheimer's Association workgroups on diagnostic guidelines for Alzheimer's disease. Alzheimers Dement 2011;7(3):263–9.
9. Sperling RA, Aisen PS, Beckett LA, et al. Toward defining the preclinical stages of Alzheimer's disease: recommendations from the National Institute on Aging-Alzheimer's Association workgroups on diagnostic guidelines for Alzheimer's disease. Alzheimers Dement 2011;7(3):280–92.
10. Sperling RA, Jack CR Jr, Aisen PS. Testing the right target and right drug at the right stage. Sci Transl Med 2011;3:111–33.
11. Bennett DA, Schneider JA, Arvanitakis Z, et al. Neuropathology of older persons without cognitive impairment from two community-based studies. Neurology 2006;66:1837–44.
12. Cummings JL, Doody R, Clark C. Disease-modifying therapies for Alzheimer disease: challenges to early intervention. Neurology 2007;69(16):1622–34.
13. Hendrix SB. Requiring an amyloid-b1-42 biomarker may improve the efficiency of a study, and simulations may help in planning studies. Alzheimers Res Ther 2011; 3(2):10.
14. Mielke MM, Wiste HJ, Weigand SD, et al. Indicators of amyloid burden in a population-based study of cognitively normal elderly. Neurology 2012;79(15):1570–7.
15. Acosta-Baena N, Sepulveda-Falla D, Lopera-Gómez CM, et al. Pre-dementia clinical stages in presenilin 1 E280A familial early-onset Alzheimer's disease: a retrospective cohort study. Lancet Neurol 2011;10(3):213–20.
16. Bateman R, Ringman JM, Rossor MN, et al. Dominantly Inherited Alzheimer Network. Clinical and biomarker changes in dominantly inherited Alzheimer's disease. N Engl J Med 2012;367(9):795–804.

17. Aisen PS, Ghetti B, Klunk WE, et al. The pathological association between Down syndrome and Alzheimer disease. Mech Ageing Dev 1988;43:99–136.

18. Campion D, Dumanchin C, Hannequin D, et al. Early-onset autosomal dominant Alzheimer disease: prevalence, genetic heterogeneity, and mutation spectrum. Am J Hum Genet 1999;65:664–70.

19. Lleó A, Blesa R, Queralt R, et al. Frequency of mutations in the presenilin and amyloid precursor protein genes in early-onset Alzheimer disease in Spain. Arch Neurol 2002;59(11):1759–63.

20. Ryan NS, Rossor MN. Defining and describing the pre-dementia stages of familial Alzheimer's disease. Alzheimers Res Ther 2011;3(5):29.

21. Fox NC, Warrington EK, Seiffer AL, et al. Presymptomatic cognitive deficits in individuals at risk of familial Alzheimer's disease. A longitudinal prospective study. Brain 1998;121(Pt 9):1631–9.

22. Klunk WE, Price JC, Mathis CA, et al. Amyloid deposition begins in the striatum of presenilin-1 mutation carriers from two unrelated pedigrees. J Neurosci 2007;27: 6174–84.

23. Ringman JM, Taylor K, Teng E, et al. Longitudinal change in CSF biomarkers in a presymptomatic carrier of an APP mutation. Neurology 2011;76:2124–5.

24. Corder EH, Saunders AM, Strittmatter WJ, et al. Gene dose of apolipoprotein E type 4 allele and the risk of Alzheimer's disease in late onset families. Science 1993;261(5123):921–3.

25. Donix M, Burggren AC, Suthana NA, et al. Longitudinal changes in medial temporal cortical thickness in normal subjects with the APOE-4 polymorphism. Neuroimage 2010;53(1):37–43.

26. Chen K, Reiman EM, Alexander GE, et al. Correlations between apolipoprotein E ε4 gene dose and whole brain atrophy rates. Am J Psychiatry 2007;164(6):916–21.

27. Burggren AC, Zeineh MM, Ekstrom AD, et al. Reduced cortical thickness in hippocampal subregions among cognitively normal apolipoprotein E e4 carriers. Neuroimage 2008;41(4):1177–83.

28. Sugarman MA, Woodard JL, Nielson KA, et al. Functional magnetic resonance imaging of semantic memory as a presymptomatic biomarker of Alzheimer's disease risk. Biochim Biophys Acta 2012;1822(3):442–56.

29. Filippini N, MacIntosh BJ, Hough MG, et al. Distinct patterns of brain activity in young carriers of the APOE-epsilon4 allele. Proc Natl Acad Sci U S A 2009; 106(17):7209–14.

30. Langbaum JB, Chen K, Lee W, et al. Alzheimer's Disease Neuroimaging Initiative. Categorical and correlational analyses of baseline fluorodeoxyglucose positron emission tomography images from the Alzheimer's Disease Neuroimaging Initiative (ADNI). Neuroimage 2009;45(4):1107–16.

31. Reiman EM, Langbaum JB, Tariot PN. Alzheimer's prevention initiative: a proposal to evaluate presymptomatic treatments as quickly as possible. Biomark Med 2010;4(1):3–14.

32. Cruchaga C, Haller G, Chakraverty S, et al. NIA-LOAD/NCRAD Family Study Consortium. Rare variants in APP, PSEN1 and PSEN2 increase risk for AD in late-onset Alzheimer's disease families. PLoS One 2012;7(2):e31039.

33. Hinerfeld DA, Moonis M, Swearer JM, et al. Statins differentially affect amyloid precursor protein metabolism in presymptomatic PS1 and non-PS1 subjects. Arch Neurol 2007;64(11):1672–3.

34. Roses AD, Lutz MW, Amrine-Madsen H, et al. A TOMM40 variable-length polymorphism predicts the age of late-onset Alzheimer's disease. Pharmacogenomics J 2010;10(5):375–84.

35. Reiman EM, Langbaum JB, Fleisher AS, et al. Alzheimer's Prevention Initiative: a plan to accelerate the evaluation of presymptomatic treatments. J Alzheimers Dis 2011;26(Suppl 3):321–9.

36. Shaw LM, Vanderstichele H, Knapik-Czajka M, et al. Alzheimer's Disease Neuro-imaging Initiative. Cerebrospinal fluid biomarker signature in Alzheimer's disease neuroimaging initiative subjects. Ann Neurol 2009;65(4):403–13.

37. Jack CR Jr, Knopman DS, Jagust WJ, et al. Hypothetical model of dynamic biomarkers of the Alzheimer's pathological cascade. Lancet Neurol 2010;9(1): 119–28.

38. Delrieu J, Ousset PJ, Vellas B. Gantenerumab for the treatment of Alzheimer's disease. Expert Opin Biol Ther 2012;12(8):1077–86.

39. Schneider LS, Kennedy RE, Cutter GR. Alzheimer's Disease Neuroimaging Initia-tive. Requiring an amyloid-beta1-42 biomarker for prodromal Alzheimer's disease or mild cognitive impairment does not lead to more efficient clinical trials. Alz-heimers Dement 2010;6(5):367–77.

40. Hendrix SB. Measuring clinical progression in MCI and pre-MCI populations: enrichment and optimizing clinical outcomes over time. Alzheimers Res Ther 2012;4(4):24.

41. Price JL, Morris JC. Tangles and plaques in nondemented aging and "preclinical" Alzheimer's disease. Ann Neurol 1999;45:358–68.

42. Markesbery WR, Schmitt FA, Kryscio RJ, et al. Neuropathologic substrate of mild cognitive impairment. Arch Neurol 2006;63:38–46.

43. Mitchell TW, Mufson EJ, Schneider JA, et al. Parahippocampal tau pathology in healthy aging, mild cognitive impairment, and early Alzheimer's disease. Ann Neurol 2002;51:182–9.

44. Guillozet AL, Weintraub S, Mash DC, et al. Neurofibrillary tangles, amyloid, and memory in aging and mild cognitive impairment. Arch Neurol 2003;60:729–36.

45. Jicha GA, Parisi JE, Dickson DW, et al. Neuropathologic outcome of mild cogni-tive impairment following progression to clinical dementia. Arch Neurol 2006;63: 674–81.

46. Grundman M, Petersen RC, Ferris SH, et al. Mild cognitive impairment can be distinguished from Alzheimer disease and normal aging for clinical trials. Arch Neurol 2004;61:59–66.

47. Alexopoulos P, Grimmer T, Perneczky R, et al. Progression to dementia in clinical subtypes of mild cognitive impairment. Dement Geriatr Cogn Disord 2006;22: 27–34.

48. Visser PJ, Scheltens P, Verhey FR. Do MCI criteria in drug trials accurately identify subjects with predementia Alzheimer's disease? J Neurol Neurosurg Psychiatry 2005;76(10):1348–54.

49. Aisen PS, Schafer KA, Grundman M, et al. Effects of rofecoxib or naproxen vs placebo on Alzheimer disease progression: a randomized controlled trial. JAMA 2003;289:2819–26.

50. Petersen RC, Thomas RG, Grundman M, et al. Vitamin E and donepezil for the treatment of mild cognitive impairment. N Engl J Med 2005;352:2379–88.

51. Jelic V, Kivipelto M, Winblad B. Clinical trials in mild cognitive impairment: lessons for the future. J Neurol Neurosurg Psychiatry 2006;77:429–38.

52. Morris J. The Clinical Dementia Rating (CDR): current version and scoring rules. Neurology 1993;43:2412–4.

53. Fox NC, Cousens S, Scahill R, et al. Using serial registered brain magnetic reso-nance imaging to measure disease progression in Alzheimer disease. Neurology 2007;69:1631.

54. Frisoni GB, Fox NC, Jack CR Jr, et al. The clinical use of structural MRI in Alzheimer disease. Nat Rev Neurol 2010;6(2):67–77.
55. Hansson O, Zetterberg H, Buchhave P, et al. Minthon L Association between CSF biomarkers and incipient Alzheimer's disease in patients with mild cognitive impairment: a follow-up study. Lancet Neurol 2006;5(3):228–34.
56. Fagan AM, Roe CM, Xiong C, et al. Holtzman DM Cerebrospinal fluid tau/beta-amyloid(42) ratio as a prediction of cognitive decline in nondemented older adults. Arch Neurol 2007;64(3):343–9.
57. Cummings JL. Cognitive and behavioral heterogeneity in Alzheimer's disease: seeking the neurobiological basis [review]. Neurobiol Aging 2000;21(6):845–61.
58. Murray ME, Graff-Radford NR, Ross OA, et al. Neuropathologically defined subtypes of Alzheimer's disease with distinct clinical characteristics: a retrospective study. Lancet Neurol 2011;10(9):785–96.
59. Wilkosz PA, Seltman HJ, Devlin B, et al. Trajectories of cognitive decline in Alzheimer's disease. Int Psychogeriatr 2010;22(2):281–90.
60. Farlow MR, Small GW, Quarg P, et al. Efficacy of rivastigmine in Alzheimer's disease patients with rapid disease progression: results of a meta-analysis. Dement Geriatr Cogn Disord 2005;20(2–3):192–7.
61. Wallin AK, Hansson O, Blennow K, et al. Can CSF biomarkers or pre-treatment progression rate predict response to cholinesterase inhibitor treatment in Alzheimer's disease? Int J Geriatr Psychiatry 2009;24(6):638–47.
62. Sano M, Ernesto C, Thomas RG, et al. A controlled trial of selegiline, alphatocopherol, or both as treatment for Alzheimer's disease. The Alzheimer's Disease Cooperative Study. N Engl J Med 1997;336(17):1216–22.
63. Courtney C, Farrell D, Gray R, et al. AD2000 Collaborative Group. Long-term donepezil treatment in 565 patients with Alzheimer's disease (AD2000): randomized double-blind trial. Lancet 2004;363(9427):2105–15.
64. Chow SC, Chang M. Adaptive design methods in clinical trials—a review. Orphanet J Rare Dis 2008;3:11.
65. Mohs K, Rosen W, Davis K. The Alzheimer's Disease Assessment Scale: an instrument for assessing treatment efficacy. Psychopharmacol Bull 1983;19:448–50.
66. Rosen W, Mohs R, Davis K. A new rating scale for Alzheimer'sdisease. Am J Psychiatry 1984;141:1356–64.
67. Cano SJ, Posner HB, Moline ML, et al. The ADAS-cog in Alzheimer's disease clinical trials: psychometric evaluation of the sum and its parts. J Neurol Neurosurg Psychiatry 2010;81:1363–8.
68. Llano DA, Laforet G, Devanarayan V. Derivation of a new ADAS-cog composite using tree-based multivariate analysis: prediction of conversion from mild cognitive impairment to Alzheimer disease. Alzheimer Dis Assoc Disord 2010;25:73–84.
69. Harrison J, Minassian SL, Jenkins L, et al. A neuropsychological test battery for use in Alzheimer disease clinical trials. Arch Neurol 2007;64(9):1323–9.
70. Gilman S, Koller M, Black RS, et al. AN1792(QS-21)-201 Study Team. Clinical effects of Abeta immunization (AN1792) in patients with AD in an interrupted trial. Neurology 2005;64(9):1553–62.
71. Perneczky R, Pohl C, Sorg C, et al. Complex activities of daily living in mild cognitive impairment: conceptual and diagnostic issues. Age Ageing 2006; 35(3):240–5.
72. Galasko DR, Bennett D, Sano M, et al. An inventory to assess activities of daily living for clinical trials in Alzheimer's disease: the Alzheimer's Disease Cooperative Study. Alzheimer Dis Assoc Disord 1997;11(Suppl 2):S33–9.

73. Galasko D, Bennett DA, Sano M, et al. Alzheimer's Disease Cooperative Study. ADCS Prevention Instrument Project: assessment of instrumental activities of daily living for community-dwelling elderly individuals in dementia prevention clinical trials. Alzheimer Dis Assoc Disord 2006;20(4 Suppl 3):S152–69.

74. Gélinas I, Gauthier L, McIntyre M, et al. Development of a functional measure for persons with Alzheimer's disease: the Disability Assessment for Dementia. Am J Occup Ther 1999;53:471–81.

75. Feldman H, Sauter A, Donald A, et al. The disability assessment for dementia scale: a 12-month study of functional ability in mild to moderate severity Alzheimer disease. Alzheimer Dis Assoc Disord 2001;15(2):89–95.

76. Mohs RC, Doody RS, Morris JC, et al, '312' Study Group. A 1-year, placebo controlled preservation of function survival study of donepezil in AD patients. Neurology 2001;57:481–8.

77. Rockwood K, Fay S, Song X, et al. Video-Imaging Synthesis of Treating Alzheimer's Disease (VISTA) Investigators. Attainment of treatment goals by people with Alzheimer's disease receiving galantamine: a randomized controlled trial. CMAJ 2006;174(8):1099–105.

78. Leber P. Guidelines for the clinical evaluation of antidementia drugs. Washington, DC: Food and Drug Administration; 1990.

79. Rockwood K, Gautheir S. Trial Designs and Outcomes in Dementia Therapeutic Research. 1 edition. Oxon. UK: Taylor & Francis; 2005.

80. Cedarbaum JM, Jaros M, Hernandez C, et al. Alzheimer's Disease Neuroimaging Initiative. Rationale for use of the Clinical Dementia Rating Sum of Boxes as a primary outcome measure for Alzheimer's disease clinical trials. Alzheimers Dement 2013;9:S45–55.

81. Doraiswamy PM, Sperling RA, Coleman RE, et al, AV45-A11 Study Group. Amyloid-b assessed by florbetapir F 18 PET and 18-month cognitive decline: a multicenter study. Neurology 2012;79:1636–44.

82. Perneczky R, Hartmann J, Grimmer T, et al. Cerebral metabolic correlates of the clinical dementia rating scale in mild cognitive impairment. J Geriatr Psychiatry Neurol 2007;20(2):84–8.

83. Schneider LS, Olin JT, Doody RS, et al. Validity and reliability of the Alzheimer's Disease Cooperative Study-clinical global impression of change. The Alzheimer's Disease Cooperative Study. Alzheimer Dis Assoc Disord 1997;11(Suppl 2): S22–32.

84. Joffres C, Graham J, Rockwood K. Qualitative analysis of the clinician interview based impression of change (Plus): methodological issues and implications for clinical research. Int Psychogeriatr 2000;12(3):403–13.

85. Walsh SP, Raman R, Jones KB, et al, Alzheimer's Disease Cooperative Study Group. ADCS Prevention Instrument Project: the Mail-In Cognitive Function Screening Instrument (MCFSI). Alzheimer Dis Assoc Disord 2006;20(4 Suppl 3): S170–8.

86. Fernández-Martínez M, Castro J, Molano A, et al. Prevalence of neuropsychiatric symptoms in Alzheimer's disease and vascular dementia. Curr Alzheimer Res 2008;5(1):61–9.

87. Lyketsos CG, Sheppard JM, Steinberg M, et al. Neuropsychiatric disturbance in Alzheimer's disease clusters into three groups: the Cache County study. Int J Geriatr Psychiatry 2001;16(11):1043–53.

88. Cummings JL, Mega M, Gray K, et al. The Neuropsychiatric Inventory: comprehensive assessment of psychopathology in dementia. Neurology 1994;44(12): 2308–14.

89. Wimo A, Nordberg G, Jansson W, et al. Assessment of informal services to demented people with the RUD instrument. Int J Geriatr Psychiatry 2000; 15(10):969–71.

90. Wimo A, Jonsson L, Zbrozek A. The Resource Utilization in Dementia (RUD) instrument is valid for assessing informal care time in community-living patients with dementia. J Nutr Health Aging 2010;14(8):685–90.

91. Wimo A, Gustavsson A, Jönsson L, et al. Application of Resource Utilization in Dementia (RUD) instrument in a global setting. Alzheimers Dement 2012. http://dx.doi.org/10.1016/j.jalz.2012.06.008. pii: S1552-5260(12)02387-4.

92. Wimo A, Nordberg G. Validity and reliability of assessments of time. Comparisons of direct observations and estimates of time by the use of the resource utilization in dementia (RUD)-instrument. Arch Gerontol Geriatr 2007;44(1):71–81.

93. Fillit H, Cummings J, Neumann P, et al. Novel approaches to incorporating pharmacoeconomic studies into phase III clinical trials for Alzheimer's disease. J Nutr Health Aging 2010;14(8):640–7.

94. Grill JD, Karlawish J. Addressing the challenges to successful recruitment and retention in Alzheimer's disease clinical trials. Alzheimers Res Ther 2010;2(6):34.

95. Edland SD, Emond JA, Aisen PS, et al. NIA-funded Alzheimer centers are more efficient than commercial clinical recruitment sites for conducting secondary prevention trials of dementia. Alzheimer Dis Assoc Disord 2010;24:159–64.

96. Thal LJ. Prevention of Alzheimer disease. Alzheimer Dis Assoc Disord 2006; 20(3 Suppl 2):S97–9.

97. Bienkowski RS, Goldfarb NM. Screen Failures in clinical trials: financial roulette or the cost of doing business? J Clin Res Best Pract 2008;4(7):1–4.

98. Knopman DS, Jack CR Jr, Wiste HJ, et al. Short-term clinical outcomes for stages of NIA-AA preclinical Alzheimer disease. Neurology 2012;78(20):1576–82.

99. Aisen PS, Petersen RC, Donohue MC, et al. Alzheimer's Disease Neuroimaging Initiative. Clinical Core of the Alzheimer's Disease Neuroimaging Initiative: progress and plans. Alzheimers Dement 2010;6(3):239–46.

Emotional and Psychological Implications of Early AD Diagnosis

Pascal Antoine, PhD[a,b,*], Florence Pasquier, MD, PhD[a,c,d]

KEYWORDS

- Emotion • Psychology • Early diagnosis • Alzheimer disease • Early-onset dementia
- Genetic screening • Caregiver • Diagnosis disclosure

KEY POINTS

Performing the diagnosis of Alzheimer disease or related disorders is considered central for high-quality care.

In patients with cognitive impairment, the diagnosis usually involves both the patient and a close relative (mostly a spouse) who will likely become the patient's caregiver, then the family and the social environment, thus changing dramatically the patient's status and role.

Early diagnosis increases the patient's empowerment.

- The disclosure situation seems to be a source of ethical conflicts that the clinician has to resolve on a daily basis.
- Early diagnosis issues are communicating uncertainty, enabling anticipation, adjusting to the patient's awareness of the disorder, not depriving the patients of their right to know, not confounding the moral pain of the disclosure with the suicidal risk, and developing one's skills for managing complex communications.
- Early-onset dementia is poorly known and consequently prone to frequent diagnosis difficulties.
- The genetic consultation is a unique support framework regarding the emotional implications associated with screening, taking into account the existential dimensions concerned by genetic issues.

Funding sources: Ministère de l'Enseignement et de la recherche.
Conflict of interest: Pr Antoine: no conflict of interest; Pr Pasquier: participated in several pharmaceutical and diagnosis trials sponsored by pharmaceutical companies, including Eisai, Ipsen, BMS, Pfizer, Sanofi, Eli-Lilly, Bayer, and Noscira, and punctually served in advisory and scientific boards for Janssen-Cilag, Eli-Lilly, Ipsen, Servier, Bayer, and Novartis.
[a] University Lille Nord de France, F-59000 Lille, France; [b] Department of Psychology, UDL3, URECA, F-59653 Villeneuve d'Ascq, France; [c] UDSL, EA 1046, CHU de Lille, F-59000 Lille, France; [d] Department of Neurology, Memory Center, University Lille, CHRU, Lille cedex 59037, France
* Corresponding author. University Lille 3, URECA EA 1059, 59653 Villeneuve d'Ascq, France.
E-mail address: pascal.antoine@univ-lille3.fr

INTRODUCTION

Previously, AD was diagnosed only at the late dementia stage.[1] Dementia was defined as a syndrome of progressive decline from a prior level of functioning, in memory and in one or more other cognitive domains, present for at least 6 months and causing significant impairment in social or occupational functioning.[2] Improvement in clinical, biologic, and imaging tools progressively made possible the diagnosis of probable AD before the late stage of full-blown dementia, at a stage in which autonomy is preserved even if some changes had appeared in the daily life of the patients, taking them to see a physician. We talk here about early AD, mild cognitive impairment due to AD,[3] or prodromal AD,[4] the borders between these terms being vague. We will not deal with the preclinical stage of AD. When the diagnosis was made at the full-blown dementia stage, the patients were barely concerned by the diagnosis and dementia was obvious for the family. The "only" shock was to disclose a disease, rejecting the simple effect of aging, and to name it, with a frightening name. We know now that AD develops for a long and variable amount of time before becoming fully apparent, and it can progress undiagnosed for years. The very first cerebral changes underlying AD probably appear 20–30 years before the first clinical symptoms. When the symptoms appear, the diagnosis can be made upon a bundle of clinical arguments[5]: subjective complaint of the patient, observation of significant changes by the family circle, medical history, neuropsychological testing, and a more or less comprehensive workup including neuroimaging and biologic tests. Still, most of the patients are diagnosed at a late stage.

The issue of an early diagnosis is far from unequivocal because it is at the crossroad of 2 distinct but interdependent phenomena: neuropathology and the experience of the patient and the entourage. In addition, it seems to be raised as an alternative to the current diagnosis, which is "late,"[5] in the sense that it is "too late" to curb or inflect the progression of the disorders and "too late" because the patients may no longer have the capacities necessary to decide for themselves the arrangements that they could have deemed as relevant. This late nature reduces the chances of getting the necessary aids and the patients' empowerment.[6] Two perspectives open up: (1) that of an *early diagnosis*, with reference to neuropathology, rendered possible simultaneously by improving the diagnostic tools and the health system, especially via the proactive screening of elderly people or (2) that of a *timely diagnosis,* with reference to the subjective experience of the disease, meeting the concerns of those who may be affected by the disease.[7] This article is in line with the latter perspective. Although the debate on the positive and negative consequences of the diagnosis of AD has been on for 2 decades, there is still a gap between guidelines and medical practices. In 2011, Alzheimer's Disease International published a report on the *benefits of early diagnosis and intervention.*[5] More recently, in February 2012, the Alzheimer's Association published an executive summary pleading for increasing disclosure of dementia diagnosis.[8]

GUIDELINES IN FAVOR OF EARLY DIAGNOSIS

The guidelines published over the past 20 years led to an increased ethical consensus on the value of the diagnosis and its disclosure. Performing a diagnosis is considered to be central for high-quality care,[9] and ethical recommendations stress the prominence of straightforward communication between the physician and the patient with regard to the diagnosis as well as the associated emotional side.[10]

THE REALITY OF CURRENT CLINICAL PRACTICE

It is estimated that about 50% of the people with a cognitive disorder receive a diagnosis.[11–13] The relatives consider than more than 2 years elapse between the first consultation justified by the symptoms and the disclosure of the diagnosis.[14] The guidelines are well known to the professionals. Nevertheless, about 50% of the clinicians aware of a diagnosis choose not to transmit the information.[12,15] The guidelines are based on a principle of autonomy and of the right to know, whereas the disclosure situation seems to be more complex (**Table 1**), a source of ethical conflicts[16] that the clinician has to resolve on a daily basis[10]: How can such news be broken without making the person more fragile? How can the patient's autonomy be respected while integrating the entourage in the diagnosis disclosure?

Table 1
Pros and Cons of the Diagnosis and Disclosure

Pros	Cons
A unique opportunity *for the patients*: • To give meaning to their symptoms • To be informed of their situation • To accept the treatment • To seek suitable help for their needs • To anticipate the needs to come • To consider inclusion in clinical research • To anticipate the future by giving their own directives about the care to implement when the alteration of judgment and autonomy may not allow for it any longer The diagnosis enables *caregivers* • To take the patient's experience better into account • To give answers to the questions and to the doubts brought about by the symptoms • To become aware of the real problem with which the patient is confronted • To obtain information on the disease (its causes, its evolution, the treatments, etc.) • To define first objectives • To participate in the treatment decision • To prepare the future on the social and financial plane • When behavior disorders are present, the entourage ascribes more easily these disorders to disease and does not question the patient himself so much • To behave appropriately The diagnosis is a gateway for orienting the clinical practices and the organization of the daily life on issues as diverse as driving a car, the decision-making process, the quality of life, or the end of life. The disclosure enables to improve the quality of life of the patients and of their relatives.	As regards diagnosis at an early stage, the symptoms may be too subtle to attract clinical attention. A diagnosis will suddenly change the status of the patients and the other people's opinion. The limited duration of the consultations may partially explain that cognitive disorders escape clinical investigation, and even when such disorders are suspected, it would be necessary to organize a follow-up so as to appreciate the evolution thereof. In such a case, the clinician considers that the knowledge of a diagnosis is really useful, especially if it may materialize with: • An appropriate way of the caregiver and the relatives to react • A therapeutic action • Coordinated home care • Or even that it does not prove deleterious to the patient. The general physicians mention several reasons for lack of diagnosis, especially: • The risk of communicating an erroneous diagnosis • The feeling of uncertainty • The feeling that the patients would rather not know • The feeling that the caregivers do not always wish the patient to be informed • The feeling that the patients could not take in such bad news • The difficulty to communicate a painful diagnosis and the associated risk of negative emotional reaction • The increase in suicidal risk

EARLY DIAGNOSIS ISSUES
Communicating Uncertainty

AD diagnosis cannot be communicated with absolute certainty, some differential diagnosis being kept in mind (including other causes of dementia). Even if improvements enable to consider a wide range of possible diagnoses among which one is AD, the criteria have still not been fully incorporated into practices and are sometimes difficult to use outside a specialized consultation, which may strengthen the feeling of uncertainty among practitioners.[17] Nevertheless, the clinician is responsible for giving information adapted to the patients on their situation. Thus, information is not imperatively a diagnosis: the physician may inform of a suspected diagnosis, explain the additional tests supposedly needed to remove this suspicion, and integrate the degree of uncertainty of the various options. The last of the 3 points is particularly important because the way the relatives understand uncertainty in the cause of the symptom is conditioned by their beliefs on the origin of the cognitive disorders.[18] Thus, the more uncertain the diagnosis, the more it is justified to take into account the patients' feeling about their situation, the understanding of the relatives to introduce a diagnostic hypothesis, and explain the reasons for the associated medical uncertainty. Such a communication is a delicate exercise, which rests on in-depth knowledge of the patient and which takes some time. This situation is potentially uncomfortable because certain patients expect from their physician straightforward information and will not be satisfied, may express their discontent, and seek a second medical opinion.

Enabling Anticipation

The relevance of informing the patient of a diagnosis in the absence of available curative treatment is sometimes questioned. The patients may be astonished or rebel against the news of their disease, and the physicians experience a difficult situation of helplessness, unable to cure. However, even if it does not lead to a curative treatment, the diagnosis is an obligatory step for introducing several aspects (**Box 1**). The topics to address during the months following the disclosure are numerous: making financial and patrimonial management arrangements, anticipating the tutorship conditions and procedures, anticipating the conditions under which daily life may become restricted (driving a car, for example), using family and professional caregivers, designating trusted people for making decisions, writing advance directives, indicating one's position regarding participation in clinical trials and research, and seeking alternatives to home support and place to live, among other issues.

None of these issues can be addressed easily, and some probably go beyond the medical sphere and the scope of the physician. Nevertheless, not communicating the diagnosis at an early stage compromises the opportunity of the patient of being

---

Box 1
Why enabling anticipation?

1. The diagnosis is a trigger, an activator of the network, both in the family and at work.

2. The diagnosis enables to offer a range of propositions among the medication treatments of specific symptoms consecutive to AD and the behavioral interventions.

3. The diagnosis is a door opened to the future: once it has been set, it is possible to anticipate the problems likely to crop up and hence to implement suitable strategies.

4. The earlier the diagnosis, the more is the patient involved in this reflection and the broader the discussion because the different parties will have had time for embracing the diagnosis.

fully involved in these decisions.[6] The observation is the same for the caregivers who report on a lack of support and information, although they acknowledge that they are not psychologically prepared to assume the caregiving role.[19] Early information increases the opportunity for the entourage to be able to take up the looming challenges. For the families, the diagnosis and its disclosure are helpful in implementing a treatment but are also factors in favor of the patients well-being. When questioned a posteriori, the families declare that they had rather known at an early stage to better react when the first difficulties appeared.[20]

Adjusting to the Patient Awareness of the Disorder

AD is characterized by cognitive disorders that may impair patients' understanding of their situation and their awareness of the existence and the extent of their disorders, also called anosognosia,[21,22] and this is particularly important because effective care for patients with AD and their relatives is related to an understanding of the extent of the unawareness displayed by the patient.[23] In the case of an early diagnosis, it may happen that insight alteration is itself an early symptom, but most often, the awareness of the disorder will be relatively preserved. Prior assessment of the patient's degree of insight would therefore be appropriate, even if it is a difficult exercise in the absence of a guide for clinical insight assessment during an interview. The physician should adopt a clear and sustainable position in the triad composed of patient, relative, and physician in the long run (**Box 2**).

The patient like the relative may seek an alliance with the physician so as to get the upper hand in growing conflicts crystallized around the reorganization of daily life. The physician plays a unique role in these triangulation situations, which are tricky to handle and provide sources of conflicts involving long-term management of communication.

Do Not Deprive the Patient of a Right One Would Wish to Enjoy

The great majority of people without cognitive alteration, including the oldest, predominantly state that they prefer to be communicated a possible future diagnosis rather than being held in ignorance,[24,25] and the same is true for patients with memory complaints attending a memory consultation.[26] Similarly, the caregivers of patients with dementia state that they would like to be informed for themselves of such a diagnosis.[27,28] This preference is in agreement with the general principle of autonomy on which is based the main ethical guidelines.[17] A posteriori, more than three-quarters of

---

Box 2
Adjusting to the patient awareness of the disorder

When insight is preserved:

The patient is able to understand the ins and outs of the situation or at least to benefit from a disclosure in a better way to be able to gradually cope with that bad news.

When insight is strongly altered:

It would be appropriate not to give up disclosing and adapting the message to what can be understood.

The necessity of reiterating the transmission of information and the exchange during the following consultations should then be anticipated, taking into account the daily difficulties of the relatives mobilized by a surveillance, which the patient, for lack of understanding, may wish to escape.

the relatives estimate the benefits of the diagnosis as quite important.[29] Only 6% consider that it would have been easier not to know. How can it then be explained that the patient's entourage is more often informed than the patient himself[30] and therefore that the guidelines that recommend giving the priority to the patient's preferences are not adhered to? The caregivers do not always wish the patient to be informed.[31] The paradox thus consists in that the caregivers wish something for themselves of which they prefer to deprive their own sick person. What is the purpose of dissimulating the diagnosis? For the relatives and the physicians,[32] the diagnostic disclosure is a situation with a risk of negative psychological reactions from the patient. This fear, and the will to protect the patient, may partially account for the resistances to the disclosure.

The Moral Pain of the Disclosure Should Not be Confused with the Suicidal Risk

Regardless of the quality of the diagnostic disclosure, it is still a disclosure of bad news, and as such, it might cause a negative emotional reaction. This reaction will be difficult to manage. The relatives already have to manage their own reaction and may not always feel able to cope with the patient's distress. The patient will experience negative feelings during the 3 months after the disclosure, in particular the fear of representing a burden for the spouse and the feeling of losing one's autonomy.[33] If this type of feeling is morally painful, its expression testifies to the integration of the diagnosis and to the patients' capacity to verbalize their feelings. In parallel, the patient will take part in the early stage of the requests for help. If the felt and expressed distress is a probable consequence of the diagnostic disclosure, the suicidal risk must be taken into account and constitutes one of the arguments opposed to the disclosure,[34] in particular at an early stage. The suicide cases of people with AD concern patients who were at the beginning stage of the disease and whose awareness of disorders was high.[35–37] However, it has not been possible to establish a link between the disclosure alone and an increase in the suicidal risk.[17] Most of the studies are retrospective and conducted in patients with a depressive episode, which may on its own account for the suicidal risk, independent of the disclosure of AD,[38,39] and the combination of other pathologic conditions such as cerebrovascular lesions or Lewy bodies may play a role.[40] The elderly people without cognitive alteration do not consider suicide as an option should they have to cope with a dementia diagnosis disclosure.[24] The prevalence of suicidal thoughts in people with dementia remains low[30] and comparable to that of the elderly people as a whole. The severity of depression before and after a disclosure did not differ in patients and their entourage, although more than two-thirds of the patients were at an early stage of the disease.[41] At the time of the disclosure, patients may first express relief that their cognitive complaints are explained and taken seriously and even express their gratitude to the specialist who confirmed the diagnosis they suspected. Conversely, the absence of diagnosis may even increase the suicidal risk.[42,43] The patients most interested in the diagnosis are the youngest and those reporting depressive affects.[44]

Developing Skills for Managing Complex Communications

The clinicians who report the greatest difficulties in initiating a diagnostic workup are those who are the most reluctant to communicate openly the diagnosis.[45,46] The disclosure of bad news is defined as a piece of information that is going to change radically and negatively the idea the patients have of their future.[47] The physician is the carrier of bad news and the witness of its impact on the patients and their entourage. The disclosure of the diagnosis of AD is a communication situation considered as one of the most difficult and stressful in the relationship between the physician and the person with dementia.[45,48] The physician is invested as the holder of the truth, whereas the reliability of the medical diagnosis is not absolute, the information received by the patient remains abstract, the information is integrated by echoing the stigmatizing beliefs associated with the word Alzheimer, and the expected concrete information (what the patient will become in the next months) is rather uncertain. Besides, the aim of the physicians, at the end of the announcement, is to mobilize the patients so that they can keep hope and face the disease. On the emotional level, the practitioners may fear the intense, unpredictable, and uncontrollable reactions of the patient and especially of the relative, to which they may feel unprepared.[47,49] Finally, the clinicians experience difficulties in finding balance between empathy, the peculiar clinical relationship, and suppressing their own emotions.[47,49]

The Factors of an Optimal Early Disclosure

Several guidelines or reviews guide the diagnosis disclosure process. In the medical field, Buckmann has suggested 6 stages for breaking bad news[47] enabling to diffuse these practices, especially in oncology. These stages have since been transposed to meet the particularities of AD.[20,50] The diagnostic process, like the disclosure itself, has a time frame, which derives from the consultation and workup delay. This duration, if it should not be too long, nonetheless permits the patients to progress in their relation with the disease and to diminish the brutality of the disclosure situation. Consequently, the approach around the disclosure should begin when the clinician has started the diagnostic process. The disclosure alone concludes the diagnostic process and ensures transition toward the implementation of the treatment and the follow-up. This disclosure is made by the specialist and relayed by the general practitioner. All at once, complying with the temporality and providing a quality link between the general practitioner and specialist are significant components.

Accompanying the Patients and Their Relatives

Well before a diagnosis can be established, it would be appropriate to know what the patients know and what are their knowledge and thoughts regarding both their current symptoms and their possible causes, among which is AD. Besides, what they wish to know and under what circumstances should be clear, in private or with their entourage. This allows to correct erroneous beliefs and to personalize the disclosure and the scheme to be implemented according to the patients' and their relatives' preferences. These interactions will enable to assess whether the people present during the disclosure will better benefit from direct than a softer approach.[27] Particular attention is paid to the ethnic, cultural, or racial differences that might influence the patients and their family understanding and preferences concerning the disclosure of the diagnosis.[51] The tests to come are generally explained in the perspective of a distinction between normal aging and a brain disease or between several diseases. The results of the tests are explained as they arrive, as the upcoming disclosure consultation is prepared, and the disclosure process is gradual over several visits.

The Disclosure Consultation

The relatives often fear the impact of such disclosure (**Box 3**) and of the word Alzheimer on the patient. However, the use of a less accurate word could confuse the patient and delay the processes of facing the reality and request for help with the dedicated services. The physicians are focused on the feelings of their interlocutors, their silences, and their solicitations, favoring the expression of these feelings and the emergence of the first questions.

Box 3
Guidelines for the disclosure consultation

1. The specialist performs the disclosure and starts with a simple and brief reminder of the consultation framework, so that the issues of the situation are clear and the patient is not flooded with information.

2. Regardless of the people present, the first questions are asked to the patients to show them who the main interlocutor is.

3. The diagnosis is given in clear and concise words, without an overuse of technical words and without any ambiguity.

4. The diagnosis must be simple and should not be too segmented.

5. It is likely that up to that stage, the exchanges with the physician were centered on the *memory (or cognitive) problems*. It is generally more appropriate once the diagnosis has been known to talk about *Alzheimer disease*.

6. The emotional load is such that the goal of the consultation should be focused on the transmission and the reception of this main piece of information.

7. The relatives report the need for a significant time for discussing the diagnosis and its implications, whereas this type of scheme is associated with the degree of satisfaction of the triadic relation (patient-physician-caregiver).

8. The rest of the consultation will enable to introduce other information, which should preferably be repeated remotely.

9. The physician explains the results of the medical tests, the immediate consequences of the diagnosis.

10. The end of the consultation is centered on the intact capacities, the short-term prognosis, the possible introduction of a treatment, and of the follow-up with a first concrete calendar.

11. In agreement with the patient, the general practitioner is informed by mail, if possible, by telephone, in the presence of the patient so that the words used are shared by everyone and the relaying process is strengthened.

Data from Refs.[17,20,50]

In the vast majority of cases, the disclosure is made to 2 persons: the patient and a caregiver. This process is a double disclosure, and the physician is hence just as attentive to the reactions of the patient as to those of the relative, seeking the participation of both. The physicians should expect a certain passivity of their interlocutors and should understand it as a form of emotional anesthesia rather than the translation of an acceptance of the disease. Time availability and empathy are mandatory. Other families will express their shock, their embarrassment of not having known about the problem at an earlier stage, or the anger of not having been heard. Cognitive focusing on the meaning of the diagnosis and its personal implications is such, as the other pieces of information transmitted, even heard, might not be taken in. A portion of the dissatisfaction reported by the families further to the disclosure probably results from the state of stupor just after the physician broke the news with dreaded words.[20]

The Consultations After the Disclosure

In the immediate aftermath of the disclosure, according to the "rule of threes,"[52] other consultations will allow to make sure that the information transmitted has been integrated and to address the evolution of the disease and the management of the possible crises. The presence of several members of the family advantageously transmits the information simultaneously to everyone and to leave everyone the possibility of asking questions on the disease and the services.[20] At a later stage, the visits will concern the use of professional helps and support groups.

EARLY-ONSET DEMENTIA

Early-onset dementia corresponds to dementia occurring before the age of 65 years.[53] Some would use the expression *young-onset dementia* when the disease occurred before the age of 45 years,[54] but both designations are confused most often. Dementia has long been closely associated with elderly or old people, and research has naturally focused on these age groups.[55] Studies on early-onset dementia remain scarce compared to those performed on older patients with dementia.[56] Better knowledge and dementia screening tools revealed a higher number of AD cases than expected in younger subjects, which raises the issue of their social recognition, of their clinical management, and of the necessity to develop research.

Dementia in younger subjects is associated with a wide variety of medical situations: AD, frontotemporal lobar degeneration (FTLD), focal atrophies, vascular dementia, dementia with Lewy body, and so forth. The most common diagnoses are AD and FTLD, and then comes vascular dementia.[55,57–59]

Early-onset dementia is poorly known, may present with atypical features, and is consequently prone to frequent diagnosis difficulties.[60] More than 70% of the families report problems associated with the diagnosis.[61] The delay before the diagnosis is long,[59,62] longer than in *late-onset dementia*[63,64] after an average of 3 clinician opinions and 3.5 years.[61] In one-third to half of the cases, the diagnosis remains uncertain and sometimes even wrong.[65] The multiplicity of possible causes of early-onset dementia, the atypical presentation of focal AD more frequently in early than in late cases, as well as the prominence of the neuropsychiatric symptoms make the diagnosis approach more complex.[60] The diagnosis is especially difficult in patients with a psychiatric history, cognitive disability or retardation, or social deprivation. All these difficulties increase the delay between the first symptoms and the diagnosis. Owing to the unenlightened representations regarding dementia, it is practically impossible for young patients and their entourage to consider that possibility, contributing to the consultation delay with the most suitable professionals. Moreover, the general practitioners, consulted as a first intent, are themselves less inclined to make such a diagnostic hypothesis for a younger patient. The first symptoms alerting the patient are often attributed to a depressive episode, a chronic stress, a professional burnout, or menopause-related changes leading to as many diagnostic errors.[66] The psychological impact of the diagnosis is especially important[67] because of the surprise of being afflicted by a disease perceived as specific to old age and the perspective of the looming deterioration.

Emotional Implications of Early Alzheimer Disease

The patients may be parents of children or of teenagers and have elderly parents themselves, in a situation of more or less important dependence. These patients often live in a conjugal relationship, with the disease upsetting the couple dynamic. The caregivers, often the spouse, confronted with a disease, which normally affects the elderly or very old people, may find themselves destitute or feel excluded, stigmatized, or socially isolated, and all this is more so in the absence of help schemes designed for them.[68,69] The onset of dementia is systematically associated with a psychological and emotional distress of the persons affected as well as of their entourage,[56] in particular in the case of young patients. These patients experience a loss of autonomy because they are not able anymore to perform the daily tasks. This increasing dependence implies a modification of the relationships with the spouse and the close and the distant family members, sometimes leading to reversal of the roles, with the children becoming the caregivers of their own parent, especially deleterious in very young adults. Moreover, if the loss of a job that one cannot take on any longer has a far-reaching financial impact, the consequences of this loss go beyond, affecting self-esteem and a whole variety of values.[53]

Psychosocial Implications of Early Alzheimer Disease

From a financial viewpoint, it seems that the cost directly associated with the disease is at least equivalent to that of later forms. However, in the case of young patients, the families have to manage the costs inherent to the disease and to informal caregiving while supporting the decrease or the loss of income. Early-onset dementia indeed affects active people whose wage represents all or in part the financial resources of the family. Consequently, the disease challenges the financial security of the family, which is not so often the case in late-onset dementia. In numerous countries, the situation of these families is financially critical because early-onset dementia may not be taken into consideration by the handicap assistance systems or by the elderly people assistance systems.

Psychological Implications of Early Alzheimer Disease for the Caregivers

A few investigations concerned the impact of early-onset dementia on the relatives.[61,68,69] These studies report that these caregivers are men as well as women[59] and are rather young,[68] most often in their fifties. The physical and emotional consequences of being a caregiver, already vastly documented regarding the families of elderly patients with AD, are also referred to by these studies, so that it is possible to compare the cases when the patient is older versus young. Some work has established, independent of the form of dementia, that the fact of being a young patient as well as a young caregiver is associated with high levels of burden.[68,70] In the case of early-onset dementia, the so-called burden measures are higher,[68] and two-thirds of the caregivers assess their level of well-being as low.[59] The intensity of distress reported by these studies was associated with the duration of the caregiving situation and by the lack of professional and informal supports for these families.[71] These investigators also assume that the lack of preparation of the families confronted with a disease, which is a priori so unlikely, would represent an additional distress factor. Several studies stressed the prominence of the emotional consequences of the diagnosis process and of the disclosure for the young patients and their family. Results emphasize the need for services centered on the person, for early identification and early diagnosis.[72] Early dementia thoroughly disturbs the individual's existence, requiring adaptive responses for maintaining their identity and quality of life.[73] Genetics explains certain forms of early dementia.[74] As gene mutations identified by predictive medicine and tests for screening are growing, although all the genes are not known and their impact not always characterized, difficulties and ethical issues can be anticipated around this practice for relatives at risk, whether they are carriers of the mutation or not.[75]

GENETIC TESTING

Studies in genetics have enabled to identify genes whose mutation or polymorphisms are considered as cause or susceptibility factors of AD. Genetic susceptibility testing is becoming a major clinical and ethical issue,[76] especially in asymptomatic people.

The first studies on the psychological consequences of the assessment of the genetic risk of AD and of its disclosure show an emotional distress associated with the bad news[77] without increased anxiety[78] but, in some patients, an increase in depression and general distress measures.[79] These studies enhance the benefits of assessing individuals' illness beliefs such as perceived risk and concern about developing the disease before, and after providing interventions that address these beliefs to facilitate test recipients' coping. Availability of preventive interventions could change the psychological consequence or genetic susceptibility testing.

Preliminary studies in healthy 50% risk relatives of patients with autosomal dominant dementias involved in a multidisciplinary protocol after Huntington disease counseling guidelines[80] did not show negative emotional reactions; no patient would recommend against performing such a diagnostic process to individuals willing to know their genetic status.[81] It was concluded that the emotional reactions were similar, although the diseases, their phenotypes, and mutations were different.[82] However, the attitudes change with increased knowledge of the disease.[83]

The genetic consultation supposedly favors enlightened decision making via preparation and education work.[84] Furthermore, this consultation is a unique accompaniment framework regarding the emotional and social implications associated with screening, taking into account the multiple existential dimensions concerned by genetic issues, the screening process itself, and the results. In AD, the practices essentially derive from the experience acquired with Huntington disease.[85] Four major axes of consultation are identified on the psychological level[86]: (1) the motivational factors that led to seek or accept screening, (2) the level of information regarding the genetic and pathologic aspects at play, (3) the level of emotional and cognitive preparation at the disclosure of the result, and (4) the level of anticipation regarding the future implications of the result (**Box 4**).

Throughout these steps, the exchanges are based on the intellectual and emotional capacities of the persons considered as integral part of a family and social background beyond their grasp.

PERSPECTIVES AND SUMMARY

It clearly seems that the current diagnosis and disclosure practices do not enable timely access to information and advice, which are mandatory for the optimum adjustment of individuals. The literature draws up an inventory of the deleterious consequences of this situation on the social, psychological, and emotional levels. This statement calls for a general reflection and perspectives in terms of research, training, and modification of practices. It should be stressed that identifying the negative consequences of the late diagnosis could not be strictly confused with the identification of the benefits of a *timely diagnosis*. Any modification aiming to correct a system could be beneficial, but should be verified, because it may introduce unexpected negative aspects to be assessed qualitatively and quantitatively. Can an earlier diagnosis really promote better acceptance of the disease and of its management? Will it enable relatives to better understand by what the patient is confronted? Will it promote real anticipation of the challenges to take on? May an early diagnosis not bring about inappropriate reactions in the entourage or in the patient? Is the suicidal risk higher in the context of an early diagnosis?

SUGGESTED RESEARCH AND TRAINING NEEDS

More than ever before, it is important to dedicate research in medical, human, and social sciences on these issues, so as to go along in real time with the changes required

> **Box 4**
> **Four psychological axes of genetic counseling**
>
> a. The aim is to assess the person's knowledge and understanding with regard to genetic screening and the links between genetics and associated diseases, as well as the meaning of their approach. This aim implies asking questions about the personal or family experience of the disease and of genetic screening and assessing motivation or on the contrary reluctance to tests. The discussion integrates the vision of the symptoms, of the alterations, of the impact on the entourage, and of the needs to come, enabling to assess the expectations and the level of understanding of the genetic approach. Thus, the persons will not only benefit from suitable medical information on screening but also be led to consider personal, family, and social questions raised by the result.
>
> b. One of the major issues of genetic consultation is learning to cope with the different steps: the test properly speaking, the expectation, the disclosure of the result, and then the future, in particular, on the case of presymptomatic testing in which the first symptoms will only appear much later. It is important to promote a preparation attitude by openly considering how to manage these different steps, the possible reactions in the face of a positive or negative result. The clinician anticipates the psychological distress during the disclosure and the necessary help strategies.
>
> c. When the person seems to be in distress, in particular during the disclosure, several themes can be involved: the feeling of uncertainty, the anticipatory anxiety, and the depressive effects. The clinician's knowledge in terms of stress management techniques, therapeutic educational strategies, behavioral and cognitive interventions, as well as professional and associative help networks provides indispensable assets.
>
> d. When it comes to genetic screening, it is important to contemplate the immediate and long-term future implied by the result. If the person is ready to engage in that exchange, the implications of his or her genetic status are discussed while taking into account the family and the financial and professional perspectives on the one hand and globally the disruption of the life choices and the existential priorities on the other hand.

by the growing scientific knowledge, the new diagnostic criteria, and the guidelines. Regarding the diagnosis disclosure, a considerable effort should be made to formalize, test, and spread training on the principles of a practice integrating uncertainty, insight, psychological distress, and communication in a situation of despair to be oriented toward a constructive anticipation dynamic. A significant research axis lies in the analysis of the interactions between the physician and the patient/relative dyad, especially the issue of emotional regulation of the actors present during the critical disclosure situation. As regards the information, it is important to promote interventions among professionals, especially general practitioners, and to facilitate access to information on the existing help networks toward the people affected by the disease. It seems important to stimulate the local professional networks, in connection with patients' associations, to work on the ethical issues raised in daily life and the progress of knowledge and changes in practices, by enhancing in parallel the communication between the specialist and the general practitioner. Indeed, if the network of help seems to develop for the patients, the physician can feel more isolated to face the challenges. Regarding the relatives/caregivers, the difficulties to which they are confronted and the importance of their caregiving role are today largely recognized. Their distress and needs are identified, and the aids and facilities for relatives are improving. Nevertheless, little work bears on a portion of the disclosure of the diagnosis to the caregivers independently from the patient. The idea is not to ignore the patients and to make decisions without involving them but to consider what the diagnosis means for the relative and to promote a debriefing time intended for the caregiver. In early-onset dementia in particular, the relatives are highly prone to distress. With the patients, they are confronted with the paradox of a diagnosis, which is all the more delayed when the onset of dementia is early. The issue, at the core of current research, is twofold: to reduce the diagnostic wandering and the resulting suffering and to promote early management, adapted to the specific psychological needs of the families. In genetic medicine, temporality is inverted: the diagnosis does not arrive at a late stage; it is the disclosure of a susceptibility, which occurs early, without being certain that the persons will effectively be ill, which will modify the vision that the persons have about their own existence. The research advances on the disease will probably move the time of diagnosis forward. The predictive validity of the indicators based on cognitive decline can be improved. Besides, biomarkers reflecting the underlying neuropathology (notably imaging, cerebrospinal fluid) take part in this evolution. The ability of these biomarkers to predict the conversion of people with mild cognitive impairments to dementia is under study.[87] It is important to develop studies on the psychological and emotional consequences with patients included in these tests, and this will provide better understanding of the experience of people early engaged in an approach suspecting neurodegenerative dementia, their understanding of the issues, and the psychological and family consequences of the result, whether they accept or not the hypothesis of a conversion toward the disease. These would be valuable preliminary data if the evolution of the approach, of a current late diagnosis, does not lead to a *timely diagnosis*, based on the optimum adequacy of the care system to the needs expressed by the patients, but to a *very early diagnosis* based on the underlying neuropathology in presymptomatic, let alone asymptomatic people. This perspective would involve totally reconsidering the diagnostic approach to integrate radically different psychological and emotional issues.

ACKNOWLEDGMENTS

This work has been developed and supported through the LABEX (excellence laboratory, program investment for the future) DISTALZ (Development of Innovative Strategies for a Transdisciplinary approach to Alzheimer disease).

REFERENCES

1. McKhann G, Drachman D, Folstein M, et al. Clinical diagnosis of Alzheimer's disease: report of the NINCDS-ADRDA Work Group under the auspices of the Department of Health and Human Services Task Force on Alzheimer's disease. Neurology 1984;34(7):939–44.
2. American Psychiatric Association (APA). Diagnostic and statistical manual of mental disorders (DSM-IV). 4th edition. Washington, DC: American Psychiatric Association; 1994.
3. Albert MS, DeKosky ST, Dickson D, et al. The diagnosis of mild cognitive impairment due to Alzheimer's disease: recommendations from the National Institute on Aging-Alzheimer's Association workgroups on diagnostic guidelines for Alzheimer's disease. Alzheimers Dement 2011;7(3):270–9.
4. Dubois B, Feldman HH, Jacova C, et al. Revising the definition of Alzheimer's disease: a new lexicon. Lancet Neurol 2010;9(11):1118–27.
5. Alzheimer's Disease International. World Alzheimer Report 2011. Available at: http://www.alz.co.uk/research/WorldAlzheimerReport2011.pdf. Accessed January 24, 2013.
6. Hamann J, Bronner K, Margull J, et al. Patient participation in medical and social decisions in Alzheimer's disease. J Am Geriatr Soc 2011;59(11):2045–52.

7. De Lepeleire J, Wind AW, Iliffe S, et al. The primary care diagnosis of dementia in Europe: an analysis using multidisciplinary, multinational expert groups. Aging Ment Health 2008;12(5):568–76.

8. Alzheimer's Association. Increasing disclosure of dementia diagnosis. In brief for healthcare professionals. Alzheimer's Association; 2012. Available at: http://www.alz.org/documents_custom/inbrief_disclosure.pdf. Accessed January 24, 2013.

9. Knopman DS, DeKosky ST, Cummings JL, et al. Practice parameter: diagnosis of dementia (an evidence-based review). Report of the Quality Standards Subcommittee of the American Academy of Neurology. Neurology 2001;56(9):1143–53.

10. Marzanski M. Would you like to know what is wrong with you? On telling the truth to patients with dementia. J Med Ethics 2000;26(2):108–13.

11. Boise L, Neal MB, Kaye J. Dementia assessment in primary care: results from a study in three managed care systems. J Gerontol A Biol Sci Med Sci 2004;59(6):M621–6.

12. Bamford C, Lamont S, Eccles M, et al. Disclosing a diagnosis of dementia: a systematic review. Int J Geriatr Psychiatry 2004;19(2):151–69.

13. Gallez C. Rapport sur la maladie d'Alzheimer et les maladies apparentées. Rapport de l'Office Parlementaire d'Evaluation des Politiques de Santé (OPEPS) 2005. Available at: http://www.assemblee-nationale.fr/12/pdf/rap-off/i2454.pdf. Accessed January 24, 2013.

14. Gibson AK, Anderson KA. Difficult diagnoses: family caregivers' experiences during and following the diagnostic process for dementia. Am J Alzheimers Dis Other Demen 2011;26(3):212–7.

15. Carpenter B, Dave J. Disclosing a dementia diagnosis: a review of opinion and practice, and a proposed research agenda. Gerontologist 2004;44(2):149–58.

16. Maguire CP. Telling the diagnosis of dementia: consider each patient individually. Int Psychogeriatr 2002;14(2):123–6.

17. Fisk JD, Beattie BL, Donnelly M, et al. Disclosure of the diagnosis of dementia. Alzheimers Dement 2007;3(4):404–10.

18. Smith AP, Beattie BL. Disclosing a diagnosis of Alzheimer's disease: patient and family experiences. Can J Neurol Sci 2001;28(Suppl 1):S67–71.

19. Ducharme F, Levesque L, Lachance L, et al. Challenges associated with transition to caregiver role following diagnostic disclosure of Alzheimer disease: a descriptive study. Int J Nurs Stud 2011;48(9):1109–19.

20. Boise L, Connell CM. Diagnosing dementia - What to tell the patient and family. Geriatrics & Aging 2005;8(5):48–51.

21. Kotler-Cope S, Camp CJ. Anosognosia in Alzheimer disease. Alzheimer Dis Assoc Disord 1995;9(1):52–6.

22. Antoine C, Antoine P, Guermonprez P, et al. Awareness of deficits and anosognosia in Alzheimer's disease. Encéphale 2004;30(6):570–7.

23. Clare L, Markova I, Verhey F, et al. Awareness in dementia: a review of assessment methods and measures. Aging Ment Health 2005;9(5):394–413.

24. Turnbull Q, Wolf AM, Holroyd S. Attitudes of elderly subjects toward "truth telling" for the diagnosis of Alzheimer's disease. J Geriatr Psychiatry Neurol 2003;16(2):90–3.

25. INPES. Perceptions, attitudes and knowledges among the general public on the subject of Alzheimer's disease. 2008. Available at: http://alzheimer.inpes.fr/pdf/en/main-results.pdf. Accessed January 24, 2013.

26. Elson P. Do older adults presenting with memory complaints wish to be told if later diagnosed with Alzheimer's disease? Int J Geriatr Psychiatry 2006;21(5):419–25.

27. Connell CM, Boise L, Stuckey JC, et al. Attitudes toward the diagnosis and disclosure of dementia among family caregivers and primary care physicians. Gerontologist 2004;44:500–7.

28. Pinner G, Bouman WP. To tell or not to tell: on disclosing the diagnosis of dementia. Int Psychogeriatr 2002;14(2):127–37.
29. Connell CM, Roberts JS, McLaughlin SJ, et al. Black and white adult family members' attitudes toward a dementia diagnosis. J Am Geriatr Soc 2009;57(9): 1562–8.
30. Holroyd S, Turnbull Q, Wolf AM. What are patients and their families told about the diagnosis of dementia? Results of a family survey. Int J Geriatr Psychiatry 2002; 17:218–21.
31. Fahy M, Wald C, Walker Z, et al. Secrets and lies: the dilemma of disclosing the diagnosis to an adult with dementia. Age Ageing 2003;32(4):439–41.
32. De Lepeleire J, Buntinx F, Aertgeerts B. Disclosing the diagnosis of dementia: the performance of Flemish general practitioners. Int Psychogeriatr 2004;16(4): 421–8.
33. Vernooij-Dassen M, Derksen E, Scheltens P, et al. Receiving a diagnosis of dementia. The experience over time. Dementia 2006;5(3):397–410.
34. Kissel EC, Carpenter BD. It's all in the details: physician variability in disclosing a dementia diagnosis. Aging Ment Health 2007;11(3):273–80.
35. Ferris SH, Hofeldt GT, Carbone G, et al. Suicide in two patients with a diagnosis of probable Alzheimer disease. Alzheimer Dis Assoc Disord 1999;13(2):88–90.
36. Lim WS, Rubin EH, Coats M, et al. Early-stage Alzheimer disease represents increased suicidal risk in relation to later stages. Alzheimer Dis Assoc Disord 2005;19(4):214–9.
37. Vega U, Kishikawa Y, Ricanati E, et al. Suicide and Alzheimer disease. Am J Geriatr Psychiatry 2002;10(4):484–5.
38. Draper B, Peisah C, Snowdon J, et al. Early dementia diagnosis and the risk of suicide and euthanasia. Alzheimers Dement 2010;6(1):75–82.
39. Seyfried LS, Kales HC, Ignacio RV, et al. Predictors of suicide in patients with dementia. Alzheimers Dement 2011;7(6):567–73.
40. Peisah C, Snowdon J, Kril J, et al. Clinicopathological findings of suicide in the elderly: three cases. Suicide Life Threat Behav 2007;37(6):648–58.
41. Carpenter BD, Xiong C, Porensky EK, et al. Reaction to a dementia diagnosis in individuals with Alzheimer's disease and mild cognitive impairment. J Am Geriatr Soc 2008;56(3):405–12.
42. Fisk JD, Beattie BL, Donnelly M. Ethical considerations for decision making for treatment and research participation. Alzheimers Dement 2007;3(4):411–7.
43. Rubio A, Vestner AL, Stewart JM, et al. Suicide and Alzheimer's pathology in the elderly: a case-control study. Biol Psychiatry 2001;49(2):137–45.
44. Jha A, Tabet N, Orrell M. To tell or not to tell-comparison of older patients' reaction to their diagnosis of dementia and depression. Int J Geriatr Psychiatry 2001; 16(9):879–85.
45. Turner S, Iliffe S, Downs M, et al. General practitioners' knowledge, confidence and attitudes in the diagnosis and management of dementia. Age Ageing 2004;33(5):461–7.
46. Cody M, Beck C, Shue VM, et al. Reported practices of primary care physicians in the diagnosis and management of dementia. Aging Ment Health 2002;6(1): 72–6.
47. Buckman R. Breaking bad news: why is it still so difficult? Br Med J (Clin Res Ed) 1984;288(6430):1597–9.
48. Cohen L, Baile WF, Henninger E, et al. Physiological and psychological effects of delivering medical news using a simulated physician-patient scenario. J Behav Med 2003;26(5):459–71.

49. Espinosa E, Gonzalez Baron M, Zamora P, et al. Doctors also suffer when giving bad news to cancer patients. Support Care Cancer 1996;4(1):61–3.

50. Derksen E, Vernooij-Dassen M, Gillissen F, et al. Impact of diagnostic disclosure in dementia on patients and carers: qualitative case series analysis. Aging Ment Health 2006;10(5):525–31.

51. Janevic MR, Connell CM. Racial, ethnic, and cultural differences in the dementia caregiving experience: recent findings. Gerontologist 2001;41(3):334–47.

52. Wald C, Fahy M, Walker Z, et al. What to tell dementia caregivers–the rule of threes. Int J Geriatr Psychiatry 2003;18(4):313–7.

53. Alzheimer's Association. Early Onset Dementia: a national challenge, a future crisis. Washington, DC: Alzheimer's Association; 2006. p. 68.

54. Kelley BJ, Boeve BF, Josephs KA. Young-onset dementia: demographic and etiologic characteristics of 235 patients. Arch Neurol 2008;65(11):1502–8.

55. Yokota O, Sasaki K, Fujisawa Y, et al. Frequency of early and late-onset dementias in a Japanese memory disorders clinic. Eur J Neurol 2005;12(10):782–90.

56. Werner P, Stein-Shvachman I, Korczyn AD. Early onset dementia: clinical and social aspects. Int Psychogeriatr 2009;21(4):631–6.

57. Harvey RJ, Skelton-Robinson M, Rossor MN. The prevalence and causes of dementia in people under the age of 65 years. J Neurol Neurosurg Psychiatry 2003;74(9):1206–9.

58. McMurtray A, Clark DG, Christine D, et al. Early-onset dementia: frequency and causes compared to late-onset dementia. Dement Geriatr Cogn Disord 2006; 21(2):59–64.

59. Williams T, Dearden AM, Cameron IH. From pillar to post - a strudy of younger people with dementia. Psychiatr Bull 2001;25:384–7.

60. Mendez MF. The accurate diagnosis of early-onset dementia. Int J Psychiatry Med 2006;36(4):401–12.

61. Luscombe G, Brodaty H, Freeth S. Younger people with dementia: diagnostic issues, effects on carers and use of services. Int J Geriatr Psychiatry 1998; 13(5):323–30.

62. Lockeridge S, Simpson J. The experience of caring for a partner with young onset dementia: how younger carer cope. Dementia 2012. [Epub ahead of print].

63. van Vliet D, de Vugt ME, Bakker C, et al. Impact of early onset dementia on caregivers: a review. Int J Geriatr Psychiatry 2010;25(11):1091–100.

64. Bakker C, de Vugt ME, Vernooij-Dassen M, et al. Needs in early onset dementia: a qualitative case from the NeedYD study. Am J Alzheimers Dis Other Demen 2010;25(8):634–40.

65. Bentham P, La Fontaine J. Services for younger people with dementia. Psychiatry 2005;4(2):100–3.

66. Harris PB, Keady J. Living with early onset dementia. Alzheim Care Q 2004;5: 111–22.

67. Pipon-Young FE, Lee KM, Jones F, et al. I'm not all gone, I can still speak: the experiences of younger people with dementia. An action research study. Dementia 2011;11(5):597–616.

68. Freyne A, Kidd N, Coen R, et al. Burden in carers of dementia patients: higher levels in carers of younger sufferers. Int J Geriatr Psychiatry 1999;14(9):784–8.

69. Kaiser S, Panegyres PK. The psychosocial impact of young onset dementia on spouses. Am J Alzheimers Dis Other Demen 2006;21(6):398–402.

70. Schneider J, Murray J, Banerjee S, et al. EUROCARE: a cross-national study of co-resident spouse carers for people with Alzheimer's disease: I–Factors associated with carer burden. Int J Geriatr Psychiatry 1999;14(8):651–61.

71. Arai A, Matsumoto T, Ikeda M, et al. Do family caregivers perceive more difficulty when they look after patients with early onset dementia compared to those with late onset dementia? Int J Geriatr Psychiatry 2007;22(12):1255–61.
72. Allen J, Oyebode JR, Allen J. Having a father with young onset dementia: the impact on well-being of young people. Dementia 2009;8(4):455–80.
73. Kinney JM, Kart CS, Reddecliff L. 'That's me, the Goother': evaluation of a program for individuals with early-onset dementia. Dementia 2011;10(3):341–59.
74. Filley CM, Rollins YD, Anderson CA, et al. The genetics of very early onset Alzheimer disease. Cogn Behav Neurol 2007;20(3):149–56.
75. Arribas-Ayllon M. The ethics of disclosing genetic diagnosis for Alzheimer's disease: do we need a new paradigm? Br Med Bull 2011;100:7–21.
76. Chung WW, Chen CA, Cupples LA, et al. A new scale measuring psychologic impact of genetic susceptibility testing for Alzheimer disease. Alzheimer Dis Assoc Disord 2009;23(1):50–6.
77. Gooding HC, Linnenbringer EL, Burack J, et al. Genetic susceptibility testing for Alzheimer disease: motivation to obtain information and control as precursors to coping with increased risk. Patient Educ Couns 2006;64(1–3):259–67.
78. Roberts S, Lock M, Prest J, et al. How does genetic testing affect anxiety about developing AD? Findings from a randomized clinical trial. Neurobiol Aging 2004; 25(Suppl 2):S509–10.
79. Ashida S, Koehly LM, Roberts JS, et al. The role of disease perceptions and results sharing in psychological adaptation after genetic susceptibility testing: the REVEAL Study. Eur J Hum Genet 2010;18(12):1296–301.
80. International Huntington Association and the World Federation of Neurology Research Group on Huntington's Chorea. Guidelines for the molecular genetics predictive test in Huntington's disease. J Med Genet 1994;31(7):555–9.
81. Steinbart EJ, Smith CO, Poorkaj P, et al. Impact of DNA testing for early-onset familial Alzheimer's disease and frontotemporal dementia. Arch Neurol 2001; 58(11):1828–31.
82. Molinuevo JL, Pintor L, Peri JM, et al. Emotional reactions to predictive testing in Alzheimer's disease and other inherited dementia. Am J Alzheimers Dis Other Demen 2005;20(4):233–8.
83. Marcheco-Teruel B, Fuentes-Smith E. Attitudes and knowledge about genetic testing before and after finding the disease-causing mutation among individuals at high risk for familial, early-onset Alzheimer's disease. Genet Test Mol Biomarkers 2009;13(1):121–5.
84. Biesecker BB. Goals of genetic counseling. Clin Genet 2001;60(5):323–30.
85. Burgess MM. Ethical issues in genetic testing for Alzheimer's disease: lessons from Huntington's disease. Alzheimer Dis Assoc Disord 1994;8(2):71–8.
86. Kaut KP. Counseling psychology in the era of genetic testing: considerations for practice, research and training. The Counseling Psychologist 2006;34(4):461–88.
87. Ballard C, Gauthier S, Corbett A, et al. Alzheimer's disease. Lancet 2011; 377(9770):1019–31.

Applying the IWG Research Criteria in Clinical Practice
Feasibility and Ethical Issues

José L. Molinuevo, MD, PhD[a,b,*], Lorena Rami, PhD[a,b]

KEYWORDS

- Alzheimer disease • Diagnosis • Biomarkers • Bioethics

KEY POINTS

- One of the strengths of the International Working Group (IWG) criteria was to reconceptualize the diagnosis of Alzheimer disease (AD), from a clinical-pathologic entity to a clinical-biologic entity.
- When a specific cerebrospinal fluid (CSF)-AD signature or a positive positron emission tomography (PET) amyloid is present in a patient, the underlying pathology is AD.
- Memory tests with cued recall measures are important to detect the typical AD hipoccampal memory dysfunction. They also present an increased capacity to predict the appearance of AD dementia and correlate with biomarkers.
- New IWG criteria applied in a clinical setting present good specificity and are feasible for the diagnosis in the prodromal stage of the disease.
- From an ethical perspective, the potential benefit of an early diagnosis may be mediated through an autonomous decision.

INTRODUCTION: THE NEED FOR AN EARLY DIAGNOSIS

In 2011, in the World Alzheimer Report titled, *The Benefits of Early Diagnosis and Intervention*, Alzheimer's Disease International discusses the importance of a timely diagnosis, as a response on patient and carer concerns,[1] and how this diagnosis should be implemented as timely as possible. A few years ago, the IWG new research criteria created a framework to establish a specific diagnosis in the predementia or prodromal

Disclosure: José Luis Molinuevo has provided scientific advice or has been an investigator or data monitoring board member receiving consultancy fees from Pfizer, Eisai, Janssen-Cilag, Novartis, Lundbeck, Roche, Bayer, Bristol-Myers Squibb, GE Health Care, GlaxoSmithKline, Merz, MSD, and Innogenetics. Dr Lorena Rami is the recipient of a Miguel Servet grant as a senior investigator from the Spanish Ministry of Science (CP08/00147).

[a] Neurology Service, Alzheimer's Disease and Other Cognitive Disorders Unit, Hospital Clínic, Barcelona, Spain; [b] Institut d'Investigació Biomédica August Pi i Sunyer (Neurodegenerative diseases group), C/Rosellon,149.08036, Barcelona, Spain
* Corresponding author. Neurology Service, Alzheimer's disease and Other Cognitive Disorders Unit, Hospital Clínic, Villarroel 170, Barcelona 08036, Spain.
E-mail address: jlmoli@clinic.ub.es

Med Clin N Am 97 (2013) 477–484
http://dx.doi.org/10.1016/j.mcna.2012.12.018
0025-7125/13/$ – see front matter © 2013 Elsevier Inc. All rights reserved.

stage of the disease.[2] The diagnosis in the prodromal stage, applying the IWG criteria, however, is considered almost experimental, because although some research supports the notion that biomarkers may help in predicting conversion to dementia,[3,4] there is yet no clear conviction that the time of AD diagnosis can be reliably advanced.[1] Although a worldwide implementation of these criteria is currently neither feasible nor desirable, the authors believe that there are several misunderstandings in how biomarkers should be interpreted from a clinical perspective, in how the IWG research criteria could be applied in clinical practice, and in the ethical background supporting early diagnosis. Therefore, this article advances and moves forward on all these matters, through revising the new conceptualization of AD, the evidence on the correlation of pathophysiologic markers with pathology, the need of a specific symptom to correctly apply the criteria and its feasibility, and the ethics of bringing an early diagnosis based in the IWG criteria into the clinical arena.

THE CLINICAL-BIOLOGIC DIAGNOSTIC APPROACH OF THE IWG CRITERIA: 2 SIDES OF A COIN

One of the strengths of the IWG criteria was to reconceptualize the diagnosis of AD, from a clinical-pathologic entity to a clinical-biologic entity. Furthermore, this approach has led to a new conceptualization of the disease, which is now considered to have a long asymptomatic period, the preclinical stage, followed by a symptomatic one.[5,6] Because there is consensus that the diagnosis should only be implemented in the clinical stage of the disease, the essence of the new IWG diagnostic criteria relies on the recognition of this dual aspect for the diagnosis of AD: a specific clinical presentation that is related to a well-defined underlying pathology. This is supported, as discussed later, by biomarkers, especially pathophysiologic markers, correlating with high sensitivity and specificity with AD pathologic features,[7,8] implying that a subject is within the continuum of the disease. Because AD pathologic changes may be already present in healthy controls,[9,10] suggesting that they are asymptomatic at-risk individuals in the preclinical stage of the disease,[5] the presence of a specific symptom, such as episodic memory deficit, is needed to certify the beginning of the clinical expression of the disease and to diagnose AD.

The Biologic Side of the Criteria

As discussed previously, the IWG set of criteria is based on a clinical-biologic approach, its biological dimension detected through biomarkers. Other articles by Blennow et al., elsewhere in this issue have discussed the specificity and sensitivity of biomarkers in establishing an earlier diagnosis and their prognostic capacity to predict future cognitive impairment. This article discusses the usefulness of pathophysiologic markers for AD diagnosis from a different perspective, their correlation with pathology, understanding that whenever there is an optimal correlation with pathology, the biomarker assessment works as a window into the brain for the diagnosing physician. Adding a specific symptomatology then confirms that the detected pathology is already expressing itself clinically, allowing an earlier diagnosis of AD.

The main pathophysiologic biomarkers are CSF markers and PET amyloid ligands. Regarding CSF, several studies have contributed to defining the diagnostic performance of CSF biomarkers and establishing a CSF biomarker signature of AD through autopsy-confirmed AD cohorts.[7,11] Because another article by Blennow et al, elsewhere in this issue is dedicated to CSF studies, this article focuses on only a few of them that are of value to confirm their utility to detect the underlying pathology.

The first study of pathologic confirmed cases to establish the value of CSF biomarkers was performed in 2008. In that study, Engelborghs and colleagues,[11] in an autopsy-confirmed sample, showed that β-amyloid 1-42 (Aβ1-42), total tau (t-tau), and phospo-tau (p-tau181P) optimally discriminated AD pathologically confirmed from controls and Aβ1-42 and p-tau181P, specifically from non-AD dementias. Furthermore, in cases of clinically doubtful diagnoses, a correct diagnosis would have been established in 14 of 16 autopsy-confirmed AD cases and a 4 of 6 of autopsy-confirmed non-AD cases, if biomarkers had been used.[12] More recently, Shaw and colleagues[7] developed, through 56 independent autopsy-confirmed AD cases and 52 age-matched elderly controls, what has been coined the CSF AD signature. In an autopsy cohort, they showed that CSF Aβ1-42 was the most sensitive biomarker for AD, with sensitivity for AD detection of 96.4%, suggesting that almost all AD cases present low CSF Aβ1-42 levels (the only one that did not show it presented CSF Aβ1-42 just above the cutoff point) and that amyloid is necessary although not sufficient to produce AD. In the same study, they also performed an analysis on the Alzheimer's Disease Neuroimaging Initiative (ADNI) cohort, showing in a logistic regression model that Aβ1-42, t-tau, and APOE ε4 allele provided the best assessment delineation for mild AD detection. In addition, an AD-like baseline CSF profile for t-tau/Aβ1-42 was detected in 33 of 37 ADNI mild cognitive impairment (MCI) subjects who converted to probable AD during the first year of the study. The investigators concluded the CSF biomarker signature of AD, defined by Aβ1-42 and t-tau in the autopsy-confirmed AD cohort and confirmed in the ADNI cohort, is able to detect mild AD in a large, multisite, prospective clinical investigation, and this signature seems to predict conversion from MCI to AD. Overall what these studies suggest is when the specific CSF AD signature is present, the underlying pathology is AD pathology.

Regarding amyloid PET ligands, the initial studies performed using PiB already showed an excellent correlation between ligand retention and amyloid plaque density in biopsy specimens.[13] The development of fluoride ligands, which are easier to use due to their longer half-lives, has culminated in recent approval by the Food and Drug Administration and European Medicines Agency of the PET amyloid ligand, florbetapir, which has shown an excellent correlation with pathology and ease of interpretation. In a recently published study, Clark and colleagues[8] compared the sensitivity and specificity of amyloid PET imaging with florbetapir with neuropathology at autopsy. In order to do it, the interpretation of the florbetapir scans, classified as amyloid positive or amyloid negative by 5 nuclear medicine physicians, was compared with the presence of amyloid pathology of participants, age ranging from 47 to103 years and cognitive status ranging from normal to advanced dementia, who were close to death. The sensitivity and specificity of florbetapir-PET imaging for detection of moderate to frequent plaques were 92% and 100%, respectively, in people who had autopsy within 2 years of PET imaging, and 96% and 100% (18 of 18; 78%–100%), respectively, for those who had autopsy within 1 year. Amyloid-assessed semiquantitatively with florbetapir-PET was also correlated with the postmortem amyloid burden in the participants who had an autopsy within 2 years (Spearman $\rho = 0.76$; $P<0.0001$) and within 12 months between imaging and autopsy (0.79; $P<0.0001$). The results obtained from this study suggest that florbetapir could be used to distinguish individuals with no or sparse amyloid plaques from those with moderate to frequent plaques. Other studies have also demonstrated the concordance of flutemetamol F 18–PET imaging with histopathology, also supporting its sensitivity to detect amyloid and potential use in the study and detection of AD.[14]

The Clinical Side of the Criteria

As discussed previously, because AD pathologic changes may be present in healthy controls,[9,10] suggesting that they may be within the continuum, the presence of a specific symptom, such as episodic memory deficit, is a central and crucial element to certify that the subject is at the clinical phase of the disease. For this reason, the IWG criteria core criterion requires the presence of an episodic memory deficit that is gradual and progressive for at least 6 months and is confirmed and reported by an informant.[2] Furthermore, in the initial article,[2] the discussion emphasized the need to properly study episodic memory, because it is considered an initial and specific symptom of AD in its typical amnesic presentation.[15] Several studies have documented the capacity of specific clinical symptoms to predict cognitive deterioration. In that sense, ADNI-derived data have shown memory deficits, measured with the Rey Auditory Verbal Learning Test or the Logical Memory test of the Wechsler Memory Scale, and FDG-PET metabolism alterations to be good predictors, in patients with cognitive impairment, of a subsequent progression to AD dementia.[16] In addition, recent studies have demonstrated that a decrease in total recall performance with tests that facilitate retrieval with cueing is highly predictive for AD[17] even at a prodromal stage.[18,19] Furthermore, in a prospective longitudinal study, Sarazin and colleagues[18] delimited specific cutoff scores for the Free and Cued Selective Reminding Test (FCSRT) that were specifically predictive of the evolution to the dementia stage of AD, even in subjects who were at the prodromal stage[18]—scores that are currently used for inclusion criteria in clinical trials. In a subsequent study performed in Germany, Wagner and coworkers[19] demonstrated that cued recall measures were more closely related to a biomarker signature of AD than delayed free recall measures, which are frequently used in diagnosing MCI. In their study, the FCSRT total recall outperformed not only FCSRT free recall but also delayed free recall measures, derived from verbal list learning (*Consortium to Establish a Registry for Alzheimer's Disease* [CERAD]) or paragraph recall, in predicting the likelihood of a pathologic CSF profile. These 2 studies confirmed the importance of using memory tests with cued recall measures, together with their increased capacity by themselves to predict cognitive impairment and correlation, with biomarkers in the prodromal AD population.

In summary, current evidence supports the use of pathophysiologic biomarkers to detect AD pathology, and cued recall tests, such as the FCSRT, for detecting an early and specific AD-related memory disorders. By themselves, biomarkers and the FCSRT have shown optimal capacity to detect AD, from a biologic and clinical perspective, thereby supporting their use together. A recent study assessing the accuracy of the current clinical criteria for the diagnosis of AD, in National institute of aging Alzheimer disease centres, shows that the sensitivity and specificity is approximately 70%.[20] By contrast, the sensitivity and specificity of PET biomarkers to detect AD pathology is above 90% and the specificity of well-assessed episodic memory performance to detect patients who will develop AD is over 90%; therefore the combination of the biomarkers plus a well assessed memory deficit is more specific and allows also to perform an earlier AD diagnosis.

TRANSLATING THE IWG CRITERIA INTO THE CLINICAL ARENA

How the IWG criteria may be implemented as a clinical-biologic approach for early AD diagnosis is discussed previously. This section discusses revising what clinical studies reveal about biomarkers and early diagnosis and discusses the authors' experience in early AD diagnosis through the implementation of the new criteria.

Although there were initials concerns about the applicability of the new research criteria, Bowman and colleagues[21] demonstrated that these criteria applied in a clinical setting presented good specificity and are feasible for the diagnosis in the prodromal stage of the disease. They found that the combination of memory impairment plus a positive CSF profile offered an optimal sensibility and specificity when applying the new research criteria. Galluzzi and colleagues[22] tried to test the validity of the new diagnostic criteria for AD in a consecutive 90 MCI patients followed for 2 years. All MCI patients with medial temporal atrophy or abnormal CSF values converted to AD being these biomarkers good predictors in this population. Prediction of AD conversion was enhanced when positivity to either medial temporal lobe atrophy or abnormal CSF was considered. The investigators concluded, therefore, that these markers are the single most robust predictors of conversion to AD in MCI patients and that their combination enhances prediction.

A recent clinical study with a long follow-up period has also contributed to defining the role of CSF markers for early AD detection. Buchkave and colleagues[4] performed a clinical study of 137 MCI patients from a memory disorder clinic with a median follow-up of 9.2 years. During follow-up, 72 patients (53.7%) developed AD and 21 (15.7%) progressed to other forms of dementia. They found that approximately 90% of patients with MCI and pathologic CSF biomarker levels at baseline develop AD within 9 to 10 years. Levels of $A\beta1$-42 were already fully decreased at least 5 to 10 years before conversion to AD dementia, whereas t-tau and p-tau seem to be later markers. A baseline $A\beta1$-42/p-tau ratio predicted the development of AD within 9.2 years, with a sensitivity of 88%, specificity of 90%, positive predictive value of 91%, and negative predictive value of 86%. These results also provide direct support for the hypothesis that in humans altered $A\beta$ metabolism precedes tau-related pathology and neuronal degeneration. It has also has to be taken into account that those MCI subjects were not specifically assessed with a cued episodic memory test, so that could be influencing the timing to develop AD.

Taking into consideration this evidence, the authors' group, Rami and colleagues,[23] tried to describe the neuroimaging characteristics of prodromal AD patients diagnosed with the IWG new research criteria, through a simplified algorithm, in a clinical setting. The relationship between neuropsychology, CSF biomarkers levels, and MRI findings was studied. In order to adapt the IWG research criteria for the study, a simplified algorithm was used, with only a pathophysiologic marker (CSF values) and episodic memory deficits as core criteria. The authors applied specific cutoff memory scores and CSF values. Prodromal AD patients fulfilling the criteria presented significant gray matter loss in brain areas traditionally associated with the initial AD pathologic changes, showing significant clusters of decreased gray matter volume in the left hemisphere regions, including the parahippocampal gyrus, uncus, precuneus, and middle frontal gyrus. Correlations revealed that prodromal AD patients with higher scores in the delayed free recall had significantly greater gray matter volume in the left superior temporal gyrus. The memory performance was also associated with CSF biomarkers levels—t-tau and p-tau levels were inversely associated with memory performance through 3 memory tests: CERAD, FCRST, and M@T (Memory Alteration Test). The posterior follow-up of these patients showed that all patients after 2 years developed AD-associated dementia, and those followed-up for only 1 year presented a significant cognitive decline. In summary, the authors observed that it was feasible to apply the IWG criteria through a simplified algorithm using specific cutoff memory scores and CSF values to diagnose AD, before dementia appears, developing in most of those patients AD dementia in the following years.

THE ETHICS OF AN EARLY DIAGNOSIS

Any medical decision generates consequences for the patient and society. Medical practice should, therefore, be performed under the guidance of the following ethical principles: beneficence, nonmaleficence, autonomy, justice, integrity, dignity, and vulnerability. Regarding the diagnosis of AD, as stated in the AD Bill of Rights, "Every person diagnosed with Alzheimer's disease or a related disorder deserves to be informed of one's diagnosis."[24] Furthermore, patient advocacy groups, such as the US Alzheimer's Association, have also been forthright on this point: "Except in unusual circumstances, physicians and the care team should disclose the diagnosis to the individual with Alzheimer's disease because of the individual's moral and legal right to know."[25]

Therefore, the major ethical issues and the correspondence ethical principles governing early diagnosis are self-determination (autonomy), efficacy (beneficence), and safety (nonmalfeasance),[26] and from the previous quotations it may be inferred that nowadays the ruling principle is autonomy, because self-determination has grown as a fundamental right of the individual, which is especially important in early diagnosis of a neurodegenerative disease, such as AD.

There is no etiologic treatment for AD, so the potential benefits of early prodromal diagnosis are to decrease the anxiety of uncertainty; to allow the early introduction of interventions, not necessarily only pharmacologic; and to help to prepare individuals and families for dementia onset. Most of these potential benefits are relative and depend in the attitude, beliefs, personality, character, and even spirituality of individuals, conferring again a primary importance on the ethical principle of autonomy. Furthermore, the psychological benefits of early diagnosis are individual related, and they may depend on a person's character, personality, and probably level of anxiety of uncertainty. In this sense, the participant applying to this kind of program and who may benefit from it most likely belongs to a self-selected subgroup of people at risk, implying a straight link with the governing principle of the program: autonomy.

Autonomy is the ethical principle related to individual freedom, personal decision-making, and self-determination. As discussed previously, it is the ruling principle of medical practice and, the authors believe, should be the governing principle of early prodromal diagnosis, because the decision of wishing to know or not to know should be performed individually by a competent individual and its potential benefit may be mediated through it. Autonomy should be reassured through self-soliciting diagnosis, permanent capacity to change one's will, confidentiality, and strict informed consent. Informed consent embodies the need to respect persons and their autonomous decisions. In this sense, competent consent is essential to justify subjects'[27] involvement in the predementia or prodromal diagnosis of AD. Competence is a pivotal concept in decision making about medical practice, allowing individuals to manifest autonomy and their right to one decides.

In the authors' experience, the will to know if a memory problem represents the beginning of AD is the main driving factor for seeking an early diagnosis. Furthermore, it is the keystone of the ethical principle of autonomy and the driver for specialists to try performing an early diagnosis on behalf of the patient's benefit.

SUMMARY

One of the strengths of the IWG criteria was to reconceptualize the diagnosis of AD, from a clinical-pathologic diagnosis to a clinical-biologic one, which can be performed in vivo. The diagnosis should, therefore, be implemented in the clinical stage of the disease, relying on the essence of the new IWG diagnostic criteria in the recognition of this dual aspect of AD: a specific clinical presentation that is related to a well-defined underlying pathology. Biomarkers measured by PET or CSF correlate with high sensitivity and specificity with AD pathologic features; episodic memory properly measured also presents high specificity to detect patients who develop AD dementia, and clinical studies have demonstrated that these criteria applied in a clinical setting present good specificity, making feasible a diagnosis in the prodromal stage of the disease. From an ethical perspective, the governing principle for early prodromal diagnosis should be autonomy, because the decision of wishing to know or not to know should be performed individually by a competent individual. Furthermore, the potential benefit of an early diagnosis may be mediated through an autonomous decision.

REFERENCES

1. Alzheimer's Disease International. World Alzheimer Report 2011: The benefits of early diagnosis and intervention. Prof Martin Prince, Dr Renata Bryce and Dr Cleusa Ferri, Institute of Psychiatry, King's College London, UK. Alzheimer's Disease International (ADI); 2011.
2. Dubois B, Feldman HH, Jacova C, et al. Research criteria for the diagnosis of Alzheimer's disease: revising the NINCDS-ADRDA criteria. Lancet Neurol 2007; 6:734–46.
3. Ballard C, Gauthier S, Corbett A, et al. Alzheimer's disease. Lancet 2011;377: 1019–31.
4. Buckhave P, Minthon L, Zetterberg H, et al. Cerebrospinal Fluid Levels of β-Amyloid 1-42, but Not of Tau, Are Fully Changed Already 5 to 10 Years Before the Onset of Alzheimer Dementia. Arch Gen Psychiatry 2012;69:98–106.
5. Dubois B, Feldman HH, Jacova C, et al. Revising the definition of Alzheimer's disease: a new lexicon. Lancet Neurol 2010;9:1118–27.
6. Sperling RA, Aisen PS, Beckett LA, et al. Toward defining the preclinical stages of Alzheimer's disease: recommendation from the national institute of aging-Alzheimer's association workgroups on diagnostic guidelines for Alzheimer's disease. Alzheimers Dement 2011;7:280–92.
7. Shaw LM, Vanderstichele H, Knapik-Czajka M, et al, Alzheimer's Disease Neuroimaging Initiative. Cerebrospinal fluid biomarker signature in Alzheimer's disease neuroimaging initiative subjects. Ann Neurol 2009;65:403–13.
8. Clark CM, Pontecorvo MJ, Beach TG, et al. Cerebral PET with florbetapir compared with neuropathology at autopsy for detection of neuritic amyloid-β plaques: a prospective cohort study. Lancet Neurol 2012;11:669–78.
9. Antonell A, Fortea J, Rami L, et al. Different profiles of Alzheimer's disease cerebrospinal fluid biomarkers in controls and subjects with subjective memory complaints. J Neural Transm 2011;118:259–62.
10. Pike KE, Ellis KA, Villemagne VL, et al. Cognition and beta-amyloid in preclinical Alzheimer's disease: data from the AIBL study. Neuropsychologia 2011;49: 2384–90.
11. Engelborghs S, De Vreese K, Van de Casteele T, et al. Diagnostic performance of a CSF-biomarker panel in autopsy-confirmed dementia. Neurobiol Aging 2008; 29:1143–59.
12. Le Bastard N, Martin JJ, Vanmechelen E, et al. Added diagnostic value of CSF biomarkers in differential dementia diagnosis. Neurobiol Aging 2010;31:1867–76.
13. Leinonen V, Alafuzoff I, Aalto S, et al. Assessment of beta-amyloid in a frontal cortical brain biopsy specimen and by positron emission tomography with carbon 11-labeled Pittsburgh Compound B. Arch Neurol 2008;65:1304–9.

14. Wolk DA, Grachev ID, Buckley C, et al. Association between in vivo fluorine 18-labeled flutemetamol amyloid positron emission tomography imaging and in vivo cerebral cortical histopathology. Arch Neurol 2011;68:1398–403.

15. Swerdlow RH, Jicha GA. Alzheimer disease: can the exam predict the pathology? Neurology 2012;78:374–5.

16. Landau SM, Harvey D, Madison CM, et al. Comparing predictors of conversion and decline in mild cognitive impairment. Neurology 2010;75:230–8.

17. Tounsi H, Deweer B, Ergis AM, et al. Sensitivity to semantic cuing: an index of episodic memory dysfunction in early Alzheimer disease. Alzheimer Dis Assoc Disord 1999;13:38–46.

18. Sarazin M, Berr C, De Rotrou J, et al. Amnestic syndrome of the medial temporal type identifies prodromal AD: a longitudinal study. Neurology 2007;69:1859–67.

19. Wagner M, Wolf S, Reischies FM, et al. Biomarker validation of a cued recall memory deficit in prodromal Alzheimer disease. Neurology 2012;78:379–86.

20. Beach TG, Monsell SE, Phillips LE, et al. Accuracy of the clinical diagnosis of alzheimer disease at national institute on aging alzheimer disease centers. J Neuropathol Exp Neurol 2012;71:266–73.

21. Bouwman FH, Verwey NA, Klein M, et al. New research criteria for the diagnosis of Alzheimer's disease applied in a memory clinic population. Dement Geriatr Cogn Disord 2010;30:1–7.

22. Galluzzi S, Geroldi C, Ghidoni R, et al, Translational Outpatient Memory Clinic Working Group. The new Alzheimer's criteria in a naturalistic series of patients with mild cognitive impairment. J Neurol 2010;257:2004–14.

23. Rami L, Solé-Padullés C, Fortea J, et al. Applying the new research diagnostic criteria: MRI findings and neuropsychological correlations of prodromal AD. Int J Geriatr Psychiatry 2012;27:127–34.

24. Black JS. Telling the truth: should persons with Alzheimer's disease be told their diagnosis? Alzheimer's Disease International Global Perspective 1995;6:10–1.

25. Alzheimer's Association website. Diagnostic disclosure. Alzheimer's Association. 2011. Available at: http://www.alz.org/professionals_and_researchers_diagnostic_disclosure.asp. Accessed June 15, 2011.

26. Beauchamp TL, Childress J. Principles of biomedical ethics. New York: NY Oxford University Press; 2001. Chapter 3.

27. Ezekiel E, Wendler D, Grady C. What makes clinical research ethical? JAMA 2000;283:2701–11.

FDG-PET in Early AD Diagnosis

Jessica Chew, BS, Daniel H.S. Silverman, MD, PhD*

KEYWORDS

- Alzheimer disease • Dementia • Prodromal diagnosis • Fluorodeoxyglucose • PET
- Progression • Multimodal imaging

KEY POINTS

- Accurate early diagnosis of Alzheimer disease (AD) helps patients to receive proper available treatment.
- ^{18}F-Fludeoxyglucose positron emission tomography (FDG-PET) is useful for detecting AD in the prodromal (symptomatic predementia) and early dementia stages, differential diagnosis of dementia, documenting cognitive decline, and predicting progression to AD.
- FDG-PET, qualified interpreters of brain scans, and imaging specialty consultation services are becoming increasingly available, and the benefits of obtaining an FDG-PET scan to determine the presence or absence of AD outweigh the costs.
- FDG-PET is a valid imaging modality to detect early AD; structural magnetic resonance imaging (MRI) may be less specific for distinguishing between neurodegenerative diseases but is needed to rule out nonneurodegenerative causes of dementia. Amyloid imaging may be useful if differential diagnosis remains unclear after FDG-PET.

INTRODUCTION

AD is the leading cause of dementia in the population older than 65 years and affects approximately 5.4 million people in the United States.[1] Although there is no cure, the ability to diagnose the disease in its early stages can help patients experience the maximum benefits of the currently available treatment options and make decisions for their future.[2]

Cholinesterase inhibitors (donepezil, galantamine, rivastigmine, tacrine) and memantine have been the only drugs for AD cleared by the United States Food and Drug Administration.[3] Although these drugs do not cure the disease, several studies have shown that prescription of these medications can delay the progression of the disease

Supported by NIH/NIA grant AG16570, UCLA Alzheimer's Disease Research Center.
Ahmanson Translational Imaging Division, Department of Molecular and Medical Pharmacology, David Geffen School of Medicine at University of California, 200 Medical Plaza, Los Angeles, CA 90095-7370, USA
* Corresponding author. Department of Molecular and Medical Pharmacology, David Geffen School of Medicine at University of California, 200 Medical Plaza, Suite B114, Los Angeles, CA 90095-7370.
E-mail address: dsilver@ucla.edu

Med Clin N Am 97 (2013) 485–494
http://dx.doi.org/10.1016/j.mcna.2012.12.016
0025-7125/13/$ – see front matter © 2013 Elsevier Inc. All rights reserved.

medical.theclinics.com

by slowing the rate of memory loss and other symptoms for some time.[4–6] As a result, prescribing these drugs in the early AD stages can allow the patients to be self-sufficient for a longer period and may delay institutionalization and caregiver needs. This benefit not only improves the quality of life for patients and their families but also helps to alleviate some of the costs of care.

FDG-PET is a biomarker for glucose metabolism that has been shown to have high sensitivity and specificity for detecting AD throughout the course of the disease, including the early prodromal stage. The Alzheimer-like hypometabolic pattern consists of decreased FDG metabolism in the parietotemporal and posterior cingulate cortices, whereas other regions such as the basal ganglia, cerebellum, thalamus, and sensorimotor cortex remain unaffected.[7] Visual analysis by expert brain PET readers has a high sensitivity to differentiate between patients with pathologically confirmed AD and other causes of dementia.[8] In addition, in recent years, numerous software programs have been developed to quantitatively analyze brain PET scans to aid visual analysis, and they can contribute to a consistently high accuracy of AD diagnosis.[9] Thus, FDG-PET can serve as a useful tool for assisting with the diagnosis of early AD.

This article discusses the multiple uses of FDG-PET in early AD, including detecting AD in both the prodromal and early dementia stages, differential diagnosis from other types of dementia, and serving as a marker of cognitive decline, as well as how quantitative methods may be able to predict progression from mild cognitive impairment (MCI) stage to AD and the future rate of decline. The article also discusses how FDG-PET compares to structural MRI and the possible reasons why FDG-PET has yet to achieve widespread clinical use for early AD diagnosis and suggests a specific way for how FDG-PET should fit into a standard clinical workup for evaluating declining cognition.

PRODROMAL AD

Under the recently revised AD guidelines, new stages of AD that precede the dementia stage have been established.[10,11] The prodromal AD stage consists of mild memory loss or onset of other common symptoms, while still maintaining a normal level of daily function. That is, it is the symptomatic predementia stage of AD.[12–14] In the clinical setting, patients with prodromal AD are those with mild decline in cognition (MDC) or MCI that are likely to progress to AD. When identified at this stage, a management plan can be implemented that may help to delay the onset and impact of dementia.

Multiple studies have shown that Alzheimer-type metabolic patterns can be found in FDG-PET scans at the prodromal stage. For example, Morbelli and colleagues[15] recently confirmed that significant FDG hypometabolism was present in the posterior parietal cortex, precuneus, and posterior cingulate cortex (PCC) of patients with prodromal AD compared with healthy controls, as determined using voxel-based statistical parametric mapping (SPM) analyses. In this study, subjects came from the European Alzheimer's Disease Consortium and patients with prodromal AD were identified as those who were classified as having amnestic mild cognitive impairment (aMCI) at the baseline time point who later progressed to AD by the end of the 2-year follow up period. The PET scans analyzed were baseline PET scans, indicating that AD can be identified at the prodromal stage through FDG-PET, which may be most apparent in younger patients with aMCI.[16]

EARLY AD

Identifying AD dementia at its very early stage is important because this is when currently approved AD medications have been found to be most effective. The characteristic AD hypometabolism in the parietotemporal and posterior cingulate cortices is evident in the early dementia stage of AD.[17]

Yakushev and colleagues[18] sought to identify early AD using automated methods and developed an SPM algorithm to differentiate mild AD from normal aging that achieved an accuracy of 91% to 100%. Meanwhile, Morinaga and colleagues[19] focused on visual analysis and found that AD-like FDG-PET metabolic patterns, visually determined by expert readers, were present in 96.7% of patients clinically diagnosed with AD at a memory clinic with a Clinical Dementia Rating of 1, the highest percentage compared with cerebrospinal fluid (95.5%), MRI (76.4%), and cerebral blood flow-single photon emission computed tomography (79.6%).

DIFFERENTIAL DIAGNOSIS

AD is not the only type of dementia that has a characteristic pattern on FDG-PET. Lewy body disease (LBD), frontotemporal dementia (FTD), and Parkinson disease (PD) have metabolic patterns that are distinctively different from those of AD. Thus, in early dementia stages when the specific type of dementia may remain unclear, FDG-PET can be a useful tool in the differential diagnosis between AD and other dementia types.

Even at the MCI or the predementia stage, AD can be differentiated from LBD on brain FDG-PET scans. The primary distinguishing feature of LBD on FDG-PET brain scans is occipital cortex hypometabolism.[20] Some LBD cases may also present with the posterior parietotemporal hypometabolism seen in AD, whereas occipital cortex metabolism is preserved in AD, making occipital hypometabolism the most characteristic feature of LBD.[21]

FTD can be differentiated from AD by unique metabolic patterns on FDG-PET.[22] Hypometabolism in the frontal lobe and/or anterior temporal cortex is associated with FTD, whereas AD is typically associated with posterior-predominant hypometabolism.[23] The differences in metabolic patterns of AD and FTD have been explored both visually[24] and using computer-automated methods.[25]

Other metabolic patterns have been found for PD, vascular dementia, and Huntington disease.[26] For patients in the predementia or early dementia stage, for which the type of dementia remains unclear, FDG-PET is an important tool that can aid in differentiating between dementia types without waiting for symptoms and the dementia to progress, allowing for earlier implementation of the optimal management plan for the patient's condition.[27]

COGNITIVE DECLINE

Beyond determining the presence of AD compared with normal aging or other dementia types, the magnitude of hypometabolism on FDG-PET also reflects the cognitive decline of patients with AD throughout the course of the disease. In the early stages, the parietotemporal hypometabolism may be asymmetric. However, as the disease progresses, the hypometabolism becomes more evidently bilateral, and in the more advanced stages, the prefrontal cortex also becomes visibly hypometabolic.[28] Lo and colleagues[29] found that glucose metabolic decline in the bilateral temporal gyrus, angular gyrus, and posterior cingulate gyrus measured by FDG-PET was significantly more rapid in subjects with AD and MCI compared with normal aging subjects over a 2-year follow-up period, whereas in the same subset of patients, more rapid decline in cognitive function was seen in those with the AD and MCI as determined by declining Alzheimer Disease Assessment Scale Cognitive Subscale (ADAS-Cog) scores. Caroli and Frisoni[30] examined the correlation between glucose metabolic rates and ADAS-Cog scores of normal subjects, patients with MCI converting to AD, those with early AD, and patients with late AD in the Alzheimer's Disease Neuroimaging Initiative (ADNI) cohort. The average level of glucose metabolism of the frontal, temporal, and parietal areas decreased as ADAS-Cog scores worsened and only reached a plateau at the very late stages of AD.[30] Thus, glucose metabolism is an indicator of the severity of cognitive dysfunction associated with AD throughout the entire course of the disease.

PREDICTING PROGRESSION TO AD

As mentioned before, AD-like hypometabolic patterns have appeared in patients who are presymptomatic or in the predementia stage. Many studies have attempted to develop automated methods to predict progression to AD in patients with predementia. Among these, Galluzzi and colleagues[31] found that 100% of 27 patients with MCI whose FDG-PET scans exhibited AD-like patterns progressed to AD after 2 years.[31] Landau and colleagues[32] determined that patients with MCI with AD patterns had a 2.7 times greater risk to develop AD than those who did not show the AD patterns. Kim and colleagues[33] found that there was more hypometabolism in frontal areas of baseline FDG-PET scans for patients with MCI who eventually developed AD,[33] whereas Morbelli and colleagues[34] found that left temporal cortex hypometabolism at baseline correlated with conversion from aMCI to AD.[34] Chen and colleagues[35] developed a hypometabolic convergence index (HCI) that automatically incorporated known AD hypometabolic voxel-based regions and was able to predict which patients with MCI would decline to AD within 18 months.[35] These studies show promise that automated quantitative analysis of brain FDG-PET scans may one day find clinical use to predict the likelihood for patients with MCI to progress to AD.

In addition to the evidence that FDG-PET can predict conversion to AD, preliminary studies have shown that FDG-PET may also be useful in predicting the rate of functional and cognitive decline. Torosyan and colleagues[36] developed a dementia prognosis index (DPI) that automatically incorporated metabolic values of cerebral regions known to be affected by AD, such as parietotemporal cortex (PTC) and PCC, and applied it to baseline scans of patients with MCI in the ADNI database. The DPI had a significant correlation to the rate of both functional decline, measured by the Functional Assessment Questionnaire (FAQ), and cognitive decline, measured by ADAS-Cog.[37] **Fig. 1** shows how the computer software used quantifies the degree of hypometabolism in AD-specific areas and the correlation between the baseline DPI and FAQ score rate of change.

MRI IN EARLY AD DIAGNOSIS

Aside from PET, structural MRI is another imaging biomarker that has been used to evaluate patients with suspected AD. MRI, like FDG-PET, is a biomarker of neurodegeneration, which in the former case is reflected by cerebral atrophy. Studies have shown that medial temporal lobe atrophy evident in MRI scans is a marker for early AD and can be useful as a predictor of progression to AD.[38,39] It has also been reported that hippocampal volume loss occurs before dementia onset and can also be used as a predictor of progression to dementia.[40] In addition, some studies have documented that the severity of cerebral atrophy is correlated with cognitive decline, indicating that MRI can also be useful to monitor disease progression.[11]

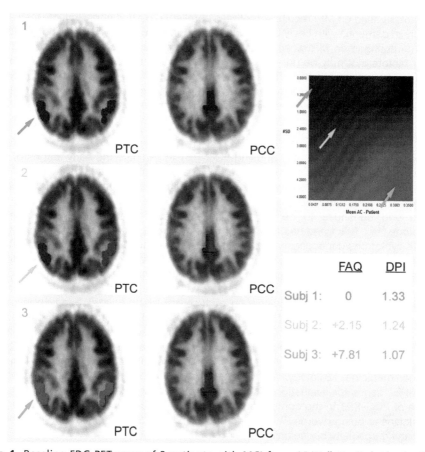

Fig. 1. Baseline FDG-PET scans of 3 patients with MCI from ADNI (http://adni.loni.ucla. edu/) using sVOI (standardized volume of interest) analysis. The top far right panel illustrates the color scheme representing different metabolic levels. Violet or indigo hues indicate very mild hypometabolism, with the color shifting toward red as greater standard deviations below the mean metabolic levels occur (*right arrow*). The top row of images show the baseline scan of a subject who had stable FAQ over 2 years (increase of 0 points/year), a baseline DPI of 1.33, and whose PTC and PCC are within normal range, indicated by the green arrow pointing to the blue of the right PTC and the corresponding location in the color scheme. The middle row of images show the baseline scan of a subject who had a mild change in FAQ over 2 years (increase of 2.15 points/year), a baseline DPI of 1.24, and whose scan shows hypometabolism in the same areas, indicated by the yellow arrow pointing to the purple of the right PTC and corresponding location in the color scheme. The bottom row of images show the baseline scan of a subject who had a large change in FAQ over 2 years (increase of 7.81 points/year), a baseline DPI of 1.07, and whose scan shows even greater hypometabolism in the same areas, indicated by the bright blue arrow pointing to the right PTC and the corresponding location in the color scheme.

However, interrater concordance for visually analyzing medial temporal lobe atrophy is low[41] and atypical presentations of AD confound interpretation.[42] In addition, despite the occurrence of dementia atrophy patterns, MRI generally is less specific for differentiating between specific dementia types, making differential diagnosis based on MRI results sometimes unreliable. Hippocampal volume loss also occurs in dementia with Lewy bodies, vascular dementia, and FTD.[43,44] Furthermore, volume changes on MRI scans that characterize dementia can also be caused by other factors that may be unrelated to dementia.[28] Overall, although MRI can serve as a useful tool to identify AD and other dementias, it may lack the specificity of FDG-PET in distinguishing between neurodegenerative conditions and finds greatest use in ruling out nonneurodegenerative causes of dementia.[44]

LACK OF WIDESPREAD CLINICAL USE OF FDG-PET FOR EARLY AD

Despite the potential benefits of using FDG-PET to evaluate the early stages of AD outlined above, it is not so widely used clinically. Reasons traditionally stated for this are the lack of availability of FDG-PET, the high cost, and the lack of expert readers. However, the availability of FDG-PET has been increasing throughout the world and continues to be on the rise, due especially to increasing use in oncology.[45,46] This trend has further led to commercial distribution of FDG, making onsite cyclotrons unnecessary. In the United States, when ordered for the indication of evaluating AD, an FDG-PET scan is only covered by Medicare for differential diagnosis between AD and FTD at the point that the patient has already progressed to dementia. Medicare has yet to approve coverage of FDG-PET for the early and prodromal stages of AD. However, a multicenter trial has also been sponsored that allows for evaluation of the effectiveness of PET information in the early stages.[47] Early detection by FDG-PET scans may lead to earlier treatments and cognitive benefits, ultimately resulting in less financial burden in the future that outweighs the initial costs of FDG-PET.[48,49] Traditionally, there has been a lack of nuclear medicine, radiology, and other physicians experienced in analyzing brain FDG-PET scans for evaluation of dementia.[45] However, with the increasing importance of FDG-PET in the context of dementia evaluations, this lack of experienced physicians is being overcome with increased training opportunities and availability of imaging specialty consultation services.[46]

ROLE OF FDG-PET IN A MULTIMODAL APPROACH

It is clear that neuroimaging will continue to play an important role in the early diagnosis of AD, and different imaging modalities have different roles to play. **Fig. 2** illustrates how MRI or computed tomography (CT), FDG-PET, and amyloid imaging can be appropriately used, based on the capabilities of each modality, in the workup for a patient whose history and physical examination reveal the presence of MDC. Structural imaging such as MRI or CT have greatest specificity for excluding nonneurodegenerative conditions such as stroke, tumors, hemorrhage, ictal activity, or hydrocephalus.[50] If any of these conditions are found on structural imaging, once they are treated, cognitive status needs to be formally evaluated. If unexplained cognitive deficits persist, or if no such conditions are found, then FDG-PET imaging should be considered after other conditions that may affect cognition (ie, depression, substance abuse, thyroid dysfunction, glucose dysregulation) have been excluded by history, physical, and laboratory examination or else have been identified and treated. The FDG-PET results will be able to reveal whether AD or another neurodegenerative process is a likely underlying cause for the cognitive complaints. However, if the differential diagnosis remains unclear after FDG-PET, and/or if conditions that may substantially affect cerebral glucose metabolism cannot be adequately treated, then amyloid imaging can be considered.[46]

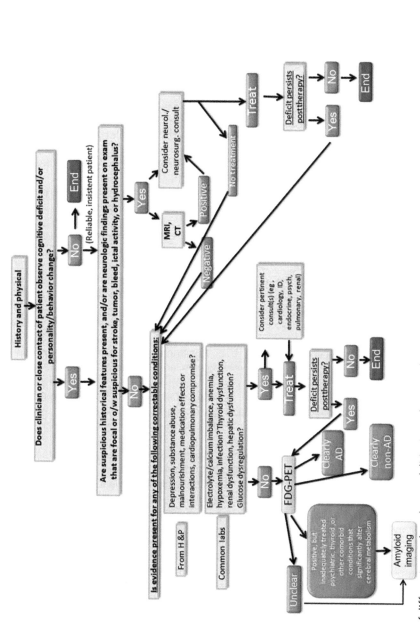

Fig. 2. The roles of different neuroimaging modalities in evaluation of mild cognitive complaints. H & P, history and physical examination; ID, infectious disease; o/w, otherwise. (*Reprinted from* Torosyan N, Silverman DH. Neuronuclear imaging in the evaluation of dementia and mild decline in cognition. Semin Nucl Med 2012;42(6):415–22.)

SUMMARY

FDG-PET is a valuable tool that will continue to aid in identifying AD in its prodromal and early dementia stages, distinguishing it from other causes of dementia, and tracking progression of the disease. As brain FDG-PET scans and well-trained readers of these scans are becoming more widely available to clinicians who are becoming more informed about the role FDG-PET can play in early AD diagnosis, its use is expected to increase.

REFERENCES

1. Alzheimer's Association. 2012 Alzheimer's disease facts and figures. Alzheimers Dement 2012;8(2):131–68.
2. Chu LW. Alzheimer's disease: early diagnosis and treatment. Hong Kong Med J 2012;18(3):228–37.
3. Galimberti D, Scarpini E. Disease-modifying treatments for Alzheimer's disease. Ther Adv Neurol Disord 2011;4(4):203–16.
4. Rountree SD, Chan W, Pavlik VN, et al. Persistent treatment with cholinesterase inhibitors and/or memantine slows clinical progression of Alzheimer disease. Alzheimers Res Ther 2009;1(2):7.
5. Wilkinson D, Schindler R, Schwam E, et al. Effectiveness of donepezil in reducing clinical worsening in patients with mild-to-moderate Alzheimer's disease. Dement Geriatr Cogn Disord 2009;28(3):244–51.
6. Peters O, Lorenz D, Fesche A, et al. A combination of galantamine and memantine modifies cognitive function in subjects with amnestic MCI. J Nutr Health Aging 2012;16(6):544–8.
7. Minoshima S, Giordani B, Berent S, et al. Metabolic reduction in the posterior cingulate cortex in very early Alzheimer's disease. Ann Neurol 1997;42(1):85–94.
8. Silverman DH, Small GW, Chang CY, et al. Positron emission tomography in evaluation of dementia: regional brain metabolism and long-term outcome. JAMA 2001;286(17):2120–7.
9. Lehman VT, Carter RE, Claassen DO, et al. Visual assessment versus quantitative three-dimensional stereotactic surface projection fluorodeoxyglucose positron emission tomography for detection of mild cognitive impairment and Alzheimer disease. Clin Nucl Med 2012;37(8):721–6.
10. Sperling RA, Aisen PS, Beckett LA, et al. Toward defining the preclinical stages of Alzheimer's disease: recommendations from the National Institute on Aging-Alzheimer's Association workgroups on diagnostic guidelines for Alzheimer's disease. Alzheimers Dement 2011;7(3):280–92.
11. Jack CR Jr, Albert MS, Knopman DS, et al. Introduction to the recommendations from the National Institute on Aging-Alzheimer's Association workgroups on diagnostic guidelines for Alzheimer's disease. Alzheimers Dement 2011;7(3):257–62.
12. Amieva H, Le Goff M, Millet X, et al. Prodromal Alzheimer's disease: successive emergence of the clinical symptoms. Ann Neurol 2008;64(5):492–8.
13. Mortimer JA, Petersen RC. Detection of prodromal Alzheimer's disease. Ann Neurol 2008;64(5):479–80.
14. Dubois B, Feldman HH, Jacova C, et al. Revising the definition of Alzheimer's disease: a new lexicon. Lancet Neurol 2010;9(11):1118–27.
15. Morbelli S, Drzezga A, Perneczky R, et al. Resting metabolic connectivity in prodromal Alzheimer's disease. A European Alzheimer Disease Consortium (EADC) project. Neurobiol Aging 2012;33(11):2533–50.
16. Kantarci K, Senjem ML, Lowe VJ, et al. Effects of age on the glucose metabolic changes in mild cognitive impairment. AJNR Am J Neuroradiol 2010;31(7):1247–53.

17. Mosconi L, Silverman DS. FDG PET in the evaluation of mild cognitive impairment and early dementia. In: Silverman D, editor. PET in the evaluation of Alzheimer's disease and related disorders. New York: Springer; 2009. p. 49–65.
18. Yakushev I, Hammers A, Fellgiebel A, et al. SPM-based count normalization provides excellent discrimination of mild Alzheimer's disease and amnestic mild cognitive impairment from healthy aging. Neuroimage 2009;44(1):43–50.
19. Morinaga A, Ono K, Ikeda T, et al. A comparison of the diagnostic sensitivity of MRI, CBF-SPECT, FDG-PET and cerebrospinal fluid biomarkers for detecting Alzheimer's disease in a memory clinic. Dement Geriatr Cogn Disord 2010;30(4): 285–92.
20. Boeve BF. Mild cognitive impairment associated with underlying Alzheimer's disease versus Lewy body disease. Parkinsonism Relat Disord 2012;18(Suppl 1): S41–4.
21. Kasanuki K, Iseki E, Fujishiro H, et al. Neuropathological investigation of the hypometabolic regions on positron emission tomography with [18F] fluorodeoxyglucose in patients with dementia with Lewy bodies. J Neurol Sci 2012;314(1–2): 111–9.
22. Foster NL, Heidebrink JL, Clark CM, et al. FDG-PET improves accuracy in distinguishing frontotemporal dementia and Alzheimer's disease. Brain 2007;130(Pt 10): 2616–35.
23. Kanda T, Ishii K, Uemura T, et al. Comparison of grey matter and metabolic reductions in frontotemporal dementia using FDG-PET and voxel-based morphometric MR studies. Eur J Nucl Med Mol Imaging 2008;35(12):2227–34.
24. Poljansky S, Ibach B, Hirschberger B, et al. A visual [18F]FDG-PET rating scale for the differential diagnosis of frontotemporal lobar degeneration. Eur Arch Psychiatry Clin Neurosci 2011;261(6):433–46.
25. Dukart J, Mueller K, Horstmann A, et al. Combined evaluation of FDG-PET and MRI improves detection and differentiation of dementia. PLoS One 2011;6(3): e18111.
26. Silverman DH. Brain 18F-FDG PET in the diagnosis of neurodegenerative dementias: comparison with perfusion SPECT and with clinical evaluations lacking nuclear imaging. J Nucl Med 2004;45(4):594–607.
27. Teune LK, Bartels AL, de Jong BM, et al. Typical cerebral metabolic patterns in neurodegenerative brain diseases. Mov Disord 2010;25(14):2395–404.
28. Johnson KA, Fox NC, Sperling RA, et al. Brain imaging in Alzheimer disease. Cold Spring Harb Perspect Med 2012;2(4):a006213.
29. Lo RY, Hubbard AE, Shaw LM, et al. Longitudinal change of biomarkers in cognitive decline. Arch Neurol 2011;68(10):1257–66.
30. Caroli A, Frisoni GB. Alzheimer's Disease Neuroimaging I. The dynamics of Alzheimer's disease biomarkers in the Alzheimer's Disease Neuroimaging Initiative cohort. Neurobiol Aging 2010;31(8):1263–74.
31. Galluzzi S, Geroldi C, Amicucci G, et al. Supporting evidence for using biomarkers in the diagnosis of MCI due to AD. J Neurol 2012;16:16.
32. Landau SM, Harvey D, Madison CM, et al. Comparing predictors of conversion and decline in mild cognitive impairment. Neurology 2010;75(3):230–8.
33. Kim SH, Seo SW, Yoon DS, et al. Comparison of neuropsychological and FDG-PET findings between early- versus late-onset mild cognitive impairment: a five-year longitudinal study. Dement Geriatr Cogn Disord 2010;29(3):213–23.
34. Morbelli S, Piccardo A, Villavecchia G, et al. Mapping brain morphological and functional conversion patterns in amnestic MCI: a voxel-based MRI and FDG-PET study. Eur J Nucl Med Mol Imaging 2010;37(1):36–45.

35. Chen K, Ayutyanont N, Langbaum JB, et al. Characterizing Alzheimer's disease using a hypometabolic convergence index. Neuroimage 2011;56(1):52–60.

36. Torosyan N, Mason K, Dahlbom M, et al. Prognostic value of PET scans for predicting rate of functional decline of normal and MCI subjects over 3 years. J Nucl Med 2012;53(S1):92P.

37. Mason K, Torosyan N, Dahlbom M, et al. Value of FDG-PET in predicting rate of subsequent cognitive decline among cognitively normal and mildly impaired subjects. J Nucl Med 2012;53(Suppl 1):461P.

38. Jack CR Jr, Petersen RC, Xu YC, et al. Medial temporal atrophy on MRI in normal aging and very mild Alzheimer's disease. Neurology 1997;49(3):786–94.

39. Geroldi C, Rossi R, Calvagna C, et al. Medial temporal atrophy but not memory deficit predicts progression to dementia in patients with mild cognitive impairment. J Neurol Neurosurg Psychiatry 2006;77(11):1219–22.

40. Devanand DP, Pradhaban G, Liu X, et al. Hippocampal and entorhinal atrophy in mild cognitive impairment: prediction of Alzheimer disease. Neurology 2007; 68(11):828–36.

41. Cavallin L, Loken K, Engedal K, et al. Overtime reliability of medial temporal lobe atrophy rating in a clinical setting. Acta Radiol 2012;53(3):318–23.

42. Galton CJ, Patterson K, Xuereb JH, et al. Atypical and typical presentations of Alzheimer's disease: a clinical, neuropsychological, neuroimaging and pathological study of 13 cases. Brain 2000;123(Pt 3):484–98.

43. Chow N, Aarsland D, Honarpisheh H, et al. Comparing hippocampal atrophy in Alzheimer's dementia and dementia with Lewy bodies. Dement Geriatr Cogn Disord 2012;34(1):44–50.

44. O'Brien JT. Role of imaging techniques in the diagnosis of dementia. Br J Radiol 2007;80(Spec No 2):S71–7.

45. Herholz K. Perfusion SPECT and FDG-PET. Int Psychogeriatr 2011;23(Suppl 2): S25–31.

46. Torosyan N, Silverman DH. Neuronuclear imaging in the evaluation of dementia and mild decline in cognition. Semin Nucl Med 2012;42(6):415–22.

47. Decision Memo for Positron Emission Tomography (FDG) and Other Neuroimaging Devices for Suspected Dementia (CAG-00088R). 2004. Available at: http://www. cms.gov/medicare-coverage-database/details/nca-decision-memo.aspx? NCAId=104. Accessed November 15, 2012.

48. Silverman DH, Gambhir SS, Huang HW, et al. Evaluating early dementia with and without assessment of regional cerebral metabolism by PET: a comparison of predicted costs and benefits. J Nucl Med 2002;43(2):253–66.

49. Moulin-Romsee G, Maes A, Silverman D, et al. Cost-effectiveness of 18F-fluorodeoxyglucose positron emission tomography in the assessment of early dementia from a Belgian and European perspective. Eur J Neurol 2005;12(4):254–63.

50. Henderson TA. The diagnosis and evaluation of dementia and mild cognitive impairment with emphasis on SPECT perfusion neuroimaging. CNS Spectr 2012;17(4):176–206.

Index

Note: Page numbers of article titles are in **boldface** type.

Med Clin N Am 97 (2013) 495–501
http://dx.doi.org/10.1016/S0025-7125(13)00038-2
0025-7125/13/$ – see front matter © 2013 Elsevier Inc. All rights reserved.

medical.theclinics.com